Non-*Helicobacter pylori* Helicobacter

-History, Biology and Disease

Second Edition

Chapters

Preface

The significance of the gram-negative, microaerophilic, spiral bacterium *Helicobacter pylori* (Hp) in the formation of gastric and duodenal diseases now widely recognized, and it is no longer necessary to explain it. J Robin Warren and Barry Marshall were awarded the Nobel Prize in Physiology or Medicine in 2005 for establishing the importance of this bacterium, which is significantly involved in gastric and duodenal ulcers. Dr. Marshall even appeared in a TV commercial that is broadcast in Japan, discussing a Meiji Dairies yogurt containing one of the lactobacilli (i.e. LG20) targeting the reduction of Hp. The Hp-based eradication of chronic gastritis has begun to be covered by the national health insurance system through the efforts of the Helicobacter Society of Japan, and approx. 1 million people receive eradication treatment each year in Japan. Gastric cancer caused by Hp may eventually become a rare disease even in Japan and east Asian countries, where gastric cancer remains a common cause of death.

However, in daily medical care, many physicians have encountered patients in whom chronic gastritis is revealed by gastroscopy, but Hp is not detected even after various tests. I have the impression that this type of case is gradually increasing now that Hp eradication has become commonplace. A polymerase chain reaction (PCR) test revealed that these cases contained a significant proportion of non-*Helicobacter pylori* Helicobacter species (NHPH), which are the subject of this book.

NHPH is included in the same genus as Hp, but has some characteristics that differ from those of Hp. Especially in terms of diagnosis, the diagnostic method that applies urease, which is widely used for Hp, often does not give a positive result for NHPH, thus overlooking these bacteria. In addition, NHPH are found not only in the mucous layer of the stomach but also in the gastric glands, especially in the intracellular canaliculus and cytoplasm of the acid-secreting parietal cells. Dogs, cats, pigs, and other non-human species are the main natural hosts of NHPH, presenting a zoonotic infection pattern. It is thus expected that the ratio of NHPH infections will increase, now that the number of people who are Hp-positive continue to decrcases due to the above-mentioned eradication, and the natural hosts of NHPH bacteria can be expected to transmit to these bacteria.

In 2010, with a grant from the Helicobacter Society of Japan, our research group began to investigate cases all over Japan by the PCR method, and we observed that a high percentage of individuals with mucosa-associated lymphoid tissue (MALT) lymphoma who were negative for Hp, nodular gastritis, and chronic gastritis were positive for NHPH. These data were reported to Helicobacter (Journal) in 2020. In recent years, as with Hp, the culturing of bacteria from biopsy tissues of dogs, cats, and humans -which was not possible in the past- has been succeeded and the whole genome analyses of NHPH have become possible. The precise infection status of each NHPH and its pathogenic factors are expected to be revealed in the near future.

In this book, we summarize or group' research history first as dialogue, and we then clarify the present challenges. The history of the research of NHPH in connection with Hp, its biology and the relation to diseases are then discussed.

Chapter 1 Looking back on our research group's 20-years history

"Why should we pay attention to this bacterium now?"

NHPH is less well known than Hp, and there are still many unclear points, especially with regard to its clinical significance. Drs. Shinichi Takahashi and Masahiko Nakamura talk about their past research and interesting points regarding NHPH.

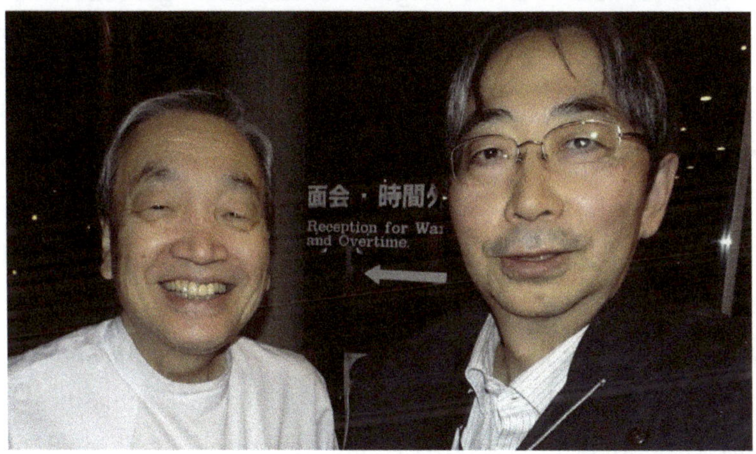

(At the entrance of Kosei Hospital, Suginami, Tokyo, Japan December 2019)

***Dr. Nakamura*:** I'm pleased to talk herein Dr. Shinichi Takahashi, vice president of Kosei Hospital-, who was the first to conduct an infection experiment on NHPH in Japan-, about the history of his research, the current situation, and future prospects concerning the clinical significance of NHPH.

In their early NHPH research, when Dr. Takeshi Ito and Dr. Takahashi infected cynomolgus monkeys with Hp, they noticed that the monkeys were already infected with another bacterium; this bacterium was reported at a Digestive Disease Week (DDW) conference, one of the largest international gastrointestinal meetings in 1994. I suspect that this was the first observation of NHPH in Japan (1). Is that accurate?

***Dr. Takahashi*:** Yes. At that time, Dr. Ito, who was at the Tokyo Metropolitan Institute of Public Health, observed a bacterium from the stomach of cynomolgus monkeys that was larger than Hp, had a spiral nature, and was morphologically similar to *Helicobacter heilmannii.* The bacterium was named *Helicobacter heilmannii*-like organism (HHLO) based on the morphological similarities. It was easy to deal with HHLO infection because it could be maintained from mice to mice in a normal environment, and used for gastric carcinogenesis experiments. However, HHLO could not be cultivated worldwide at that time.

***Nakamura*:** We have been conducting joint research on NHPH at Kyorin University (Mitaka) and the Kitasato Institute (Tokyo) for over 20 years - since 2000. Initial perception was that these bacteria were spiral and stronger than Hp in C3H mice, but Dr. Somay Y Murayama clarified that NHPH bacteria HHLOs, based on the analysis of 16S rDNA and the detailed sequence. The bacteria were first thought to belong to *H. heilmannii ss (sensu stricto)* at the beginning and *H. suis* in subsequent analyses and reported to the journal *Infection Immunity* in 2006. At that time, the connection between these bacteria and clinical observations was not clear, and we did not get much interest in our findings among clinicians.

***Takahashi*:** Shortly before that, Professor Akifumi Tanaka from Kyorin University began a research study at Shinshu University (Nagano, Japan), and Professors Hiroyoshi Ota and Tsutomu Katsuyama of Shinshu University and other physicians and researchers identified many NHPH-positive cases there.

***Nakamura*:** Another discovery in this connection was the formation of gastric MALT lymphoma in an infection experiment. As part of my involvement with students' graduation theses as a member of the Faculty of Pharmacy, Kitasato University (Tokyo, Japan), an experiment was conducted to infect C57BL / 6 mice from C3H mice with NHPH, but only mild gastritis was formed in the C3H mice, whereas the C57BL/6 mice developed marked lymphocyte aggregation in the gastric mucosa, i.e. lymph follicle formation. The difference was so striking with hematoxylin-eosin (H&E) staining that, I contacted the student in charge of the experiment, he responded, "Did you make a mistake? "

***Takahashi*:** Physicians and researchers from Kyorin University, Kitasato University, and Shinshu University gathered to hold an NHPH study group meeting twice a year in Tokyo and Matsumoto alternately from 2006 to 2008, and a considerable amount of data were accumulated. Professor Shoko Nakazawa (Yamaguchi University [Yamaguchi, Japan] at that time), who participated as the special guest, provided us with a great deal of bacteriology information, and at the post-study social gathering, the discussions continued with enthusiasm, leaving everyone highly excited to lead the world in NHPH research.

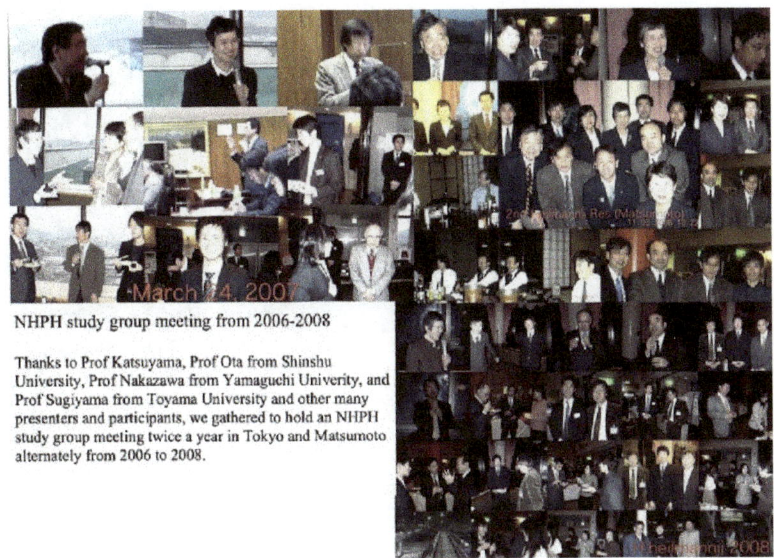

NHPH study group meeting from 2006-2008

Thanks to Prof Katsuyama, Prof Ota from Shinshu University, Prof Nakazawa from Yamaguchi Univerity, and Prof Sugiyama from Toyama University and other many presenters and participants, we gathered to hold an NHPH study group meeting twice a year in Tokyo and Matsumoto alternately from 2006 to 2008.

***Nakamura*:** We also held three international symposiums. The first meeting was held in April 2007, and we invited Professor Jani O'Rourke of New South Wales University in Australia. She reported the phylogenetic trec of NHPH based on analyses of the stomachs of animals at Sydney's famous Taronga Zoo. Those studies were undertaken under Dr. Adrian Lee, who laid the foundation for basic research on Hp.

International Symposium on Helicobacter heilmannii
April 25, 2007 (Kitasato University)

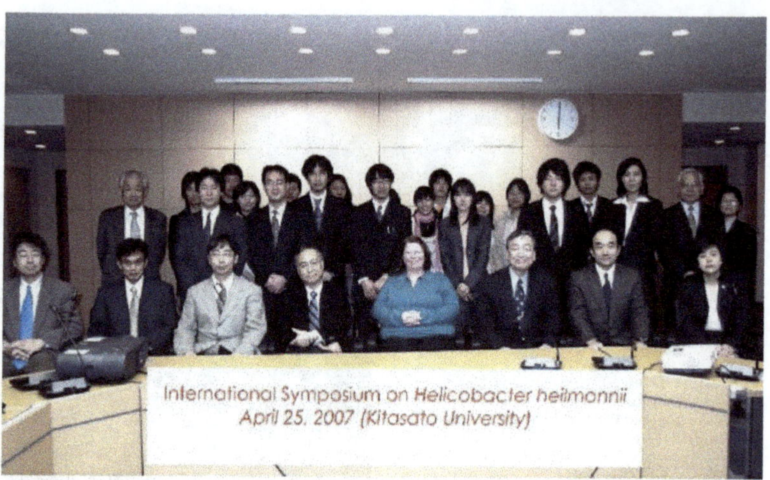

APRIL 2007 *Dr O'Rourke visited our laboratory and held an international symposium.*

The second meeting was held in April 2009, and we invited Dr. Hazel Mitchel from New South Wales University, the same facility as Dr. O'Rourke. She reported the relationship between colorectal diseases and NHPH.

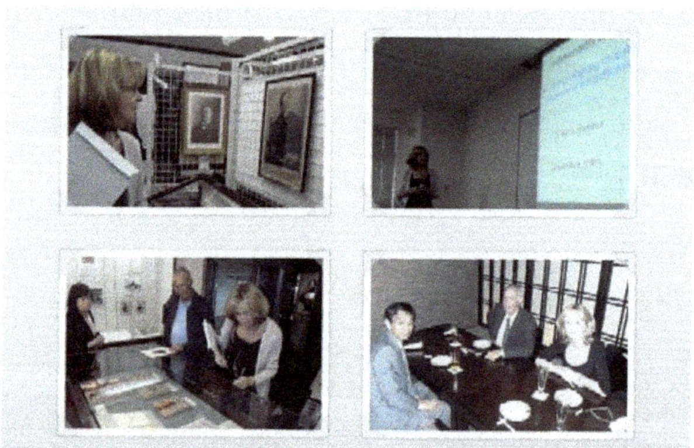

The third meeting was held in June 2015, and Dr. Bram Flahou of Ghent University in Belgium joined us. Under the supervision of Dr. Freddy Hausebrouck, a well-known researcher in the field of veterinary medicine, he succeeded in isolating and culturing various types of NHPHs from dogs and cats using a new method. Anders Øverby, who came from NTNU (Norwegian University of Science and Technology) and studied in our laboratory at that time, learned the new method, and succeeded in culturing *Helicobacter heilmannii ss* derived from cats, and reported on its bacteriological characteristics.

3rd International Consensus Symposium on
Helicobacter heilmannii/suis June 29, 2015

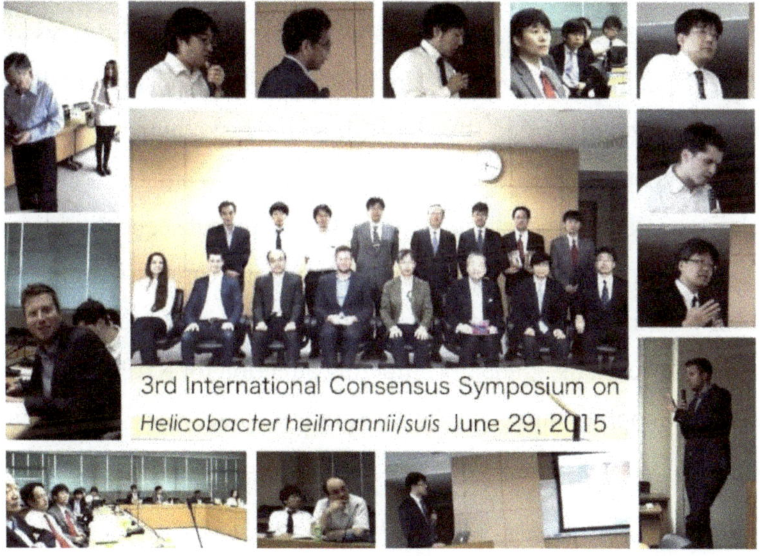

***Takahashi*:** The 2015 symposium was fun and fruitful, as we had fascinating discussions with researchers from all over the world and asked many questions. It was great occasion to learn about the context of our research in the world and to think about future issues. I was surprised and grateful to Professor Nakamura for holding such a study group.

***Nakamura*:** Thank you. A nationwide survey of clinical cases in Japan with a grant from the Helicobacter Society of Japan was recently published in the journal *Helicobacter*. Although it took time, we were able to analyze a large number of cases, and we are grateful to gastroenterologists all over Japan for their cooperation. Concerning nodular gastritis, we were able to analyze dozens of NHPH-positive cases. The first case of NHPH-positive nodular gastritis was reported by Dr. Shinichi Nakamura, from the Department of Gastroenterology, Tokyo Women's Medical University and this bacterium has been used for subsequent analysis. In addition, physicians and researchers from various institutions with whom we have collaborated have made many presentations in academic journals, gradually attracting attention for NHPHs. We've also had opportunities to be featured in magazines for public audiences.

***Takahashi*:** Unlike Hp, NHPH would not obtain much interest if it were not related to human diseases. Dr. Nakamura inoculated mice with NHPH strains from cynomolgus monkey and human to develop gastric MALT lymphoma, which has been prevalent in Asia. The eradication of NHPH and pharmacological treatments of MALT lymphoma have been used for humans, and are thus of interest to many clinicians. NHPH has been taken up as a theme subject at academic societies. I'm looking forward to future studies.

***Nakamura*:** Based on your many years research of Hp, what do you think we should pay attention in future research?

***Takahashi*:** First, looking back on the history of Hp research, it should be noted that Dr. Warren first discovered it in the gastric mucosa of a gastritis patient by a microscopic examination, and then Dr. Marshall succeeded in culturing the bacterium; they were then able to see link between their findings and many clinical cases. Many randomized control trials later demonstrated the efficacy of Hp eradication to prevent the recurrence of peptic ulcer, and research has elucidated the ability of Hp eradication to improve chronic active gastritis and reducing the number of gastric cancer deaths. Similarly, for NHPH, the establishment of a diagnostic method is fundamental. I think it is necessary to confirm the infection status nationwide everywhere that it is possible to do so, determine the etiologic relationship between NHPH and various diseases, and develop effective eradication methods. As a researcher, one is always aware that many ‘unknowns’ remain, and I think we will continue to find this field of research even more compelling.

***Nakamura*:** Thank you. We look forward to your continued guidance in the future.

Chapter 2 History of gastric NHPH researc

The history of research on gastric NHPH can be traced to long before the discovery of *Helicobacter pylori* - shortly after the discovery of the microscope, in fact. However, it is only recently that the association between NHPH and lesion formation has come to the fore.

1. Koch's four postulates

The discovery of Hp is generally said to have been by Warren, Marshall in 1983, but many spiral bacteria were observed in the mammalian stomach before that. Warren and Marshall are given credit for not only identifying Hp, but also satisfying Robert Koch's four postulates: culture, infection with the bacterium, lesion formation and re-isolation of the same bacterium (Fig. 1). Although the number of bacteria species that can be purely cultivated are rather a minority among the many thousands of bacteria species, and it has recently become possible to perform gene analyses even for bacteria that cannot be cultivated.

Fig. 1 Koch's four postulates

Koch's Postulates as We Know Them Today

1. The same organism must be present in every case of the disease.
2. The organism must be isolated from the diseased host and grown in pure culture.
3. The isolate must cause the disease, when inoculated into a healthy, susceptible animal.
4. The organism must be reisolated from the inoculated, diseased animal.

Many of the spiral bacteria that inhabit the stomach of animals that have been examined since the 19th century are thought to have been gastric NHPH, rather than Hp. Unlike Hp, which was successfully cultured by Warren and Marshall, it has only recently become possible to cultivate some of the gastric NHPHs mentioned herein, by means of a two-layer culture or related procedure. First, let's examine the discoveries of Hp and gastric NHPH and the context.

2. From the beginning of the 19th century to 1917

Table 1 History of gastric mucosal spiral bacterium research from 1838 to 1917

Pre/Post	Year	First Author	Points	Hp/NHPH/others	Ref Number
		Until this time	The stomach was thought to be aseptic and supposed to be protected bygastric bactericidal barrier.		
	1838	C.G.Ehrenburg	observed spiral organism in animal gastroitestinal tract		3
	1875	G. Bottcher, M. Letulle	discoved bacteria in ulcer bed and margin		4
	1881	J.P. Rappin	detected spiral organism in dog stomach	NHPH	5
	1881	C. Klebs	found bacteria and cellular infiltration between the gastric glands		
	1888	M. Letulle	production of experimental acute gastric mucosal lesion by S Staphylococus aureus infection in guinea pig	Staphylococcus aureus	
	1889	W. Jaworski	discovered spiral bacteria in gastric gavage (in Polish)	Vibrio rugala	6
	1893	G. Bizzozero, C. Golgi	identified Spirohete in dog gastric mucosa, successful infection experiment, bacteria in gastric glandular lumen and parietal cell cytoplasm	NHPH	7
	1896	H. Salomon	discovered Spirocheta in dog, cat, rat and other animals, experimental infection to mouse. found invasion to parietal cells, failed in culture	NHPH	8
	1898	K. Shiga	reported Shigella dysenteriae interaction in gastrointestinal inflammation (wrong announcement)		
Pre-Hp		この頃	thought anthrax related to ulcer formation, but culture unsuccessful		
	1904	I.P. Pavlov	selected as a Nobel laureate by the experiment using gastric pouch showing the importance of gastric acid		
	1905	F. Riegel	Gastric ulcer was thought to derive from hyperacidity. Schwarz's maxim "no acid, no ulcer"		
	1906	W. Krienitz	found three kinds of Spirohete in gastric juice of gastric cancer patients	Hp (?)	
	1906	A. Balfour	found spiral organism near mammalian gastric ulcer	NHPH	
	1908	F.B. Turck	produced ulcer in dog stomach by E. coli, and foud E. coli in the stool of gastric ulcer patient	E.coli	
	1909	P. Carnot, A. Lelievre	denied the bacteria in parietal cell bySalomon, and insisted on effect ofgastric secretion		
	1909	C. Regaud	proved the spiral organism in the parietal cell and named as Spirochete regaudi	NHPH (Spirochete regaudi)	
	1916	E.C. Rosenow	produced gastric ulcer by Streptococcus, and postulated tooth caries as bacterial reservoir	Streptococcus	
	1917	L.R. Dragstedt	identified bacteria by experimental ulcer, but it significance was unknown. Investigated the role of vagal nerve	Streptococcus	

Hp
NHPH

Research on bacteria under a light microscope began in the 17th century after Robert Hooke – the originator of Hooke's law of springs-, published a sketch of his observations of microorganisms under a microscope. Antonie van Leewenhoek (of the Netherlands), whom Hooke introduced to the Royal Society of England, achieved a magnification of 200-plus times more with a microscope with a single lens that he polished himself. Van Leewenhoek proposed the use of the German term 'Zelle' (cell in English) to indicate a biological unit. He also described the morphology of microorganisms in the oral cavity (Fig. 2).

Fig. 2 Types of bacteria drawn by van Leewenhoek

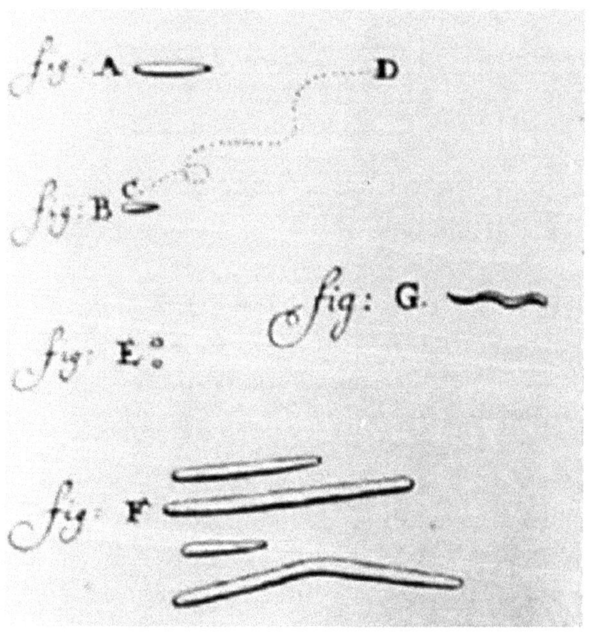

In 1786, the Danish naturalist Otto Müller observed microorganisms and coined the term "bacillus' (2). However, it was not until the 19th century that the microscopes progressed to the present combination of multiple lenses, and until the early 19th century, the stomach was considered sterile or with very few bacteria, and a so-called 'gastric bactericidal barrier' was thought to exist. The first report of spiral bacteria was by the German naturalist Christian Ehrenberg in 1838 (3). Bottcher and Letulle later detected a bacterial population on the bottom and margin of gastric ulcers in animals (4). Rappin also described a spiral bacterium in the stomach of dogs in 1881 (5). Jaworski first reported the presence of spiral bacteria in the wash solution of the stomach (6). By this time, the involvement of staphylococci, lactobacilli, pneumococci, diphtheria toxins, etc. was also being investigated, and the hypothesis that bacterial infections were at least a secondary cause of gastroduodenal ulcer was established.

Giulio Bizzozero (7) in 1892 and Salmon (8) in 1896 reported spiral bacteria in the stomach of dogs and mammals. Bizzozero reported a large number of spiral bacteria in the gastric glandular lumen and the intracytoplasmic canaliculi and vesicles of the parietal cells of the cat stomach. He instructed his subordinate Camillo Golgi, who developed the silver impregnation method as a nerve staining method and was awarded the Nobel Prize in 1906, to stain the bacteria using that method. Three years later, Salomon found spiral bacteria in the stomachs of dogs, cats and rats, and succeeded in infecting mice (Fig. 3).

Fig. 3 Distribution of canine-derived spiral bacteria in the mouse stomach by Salomon. An aggregation of bacteria is observed in the mucus layer and in the gastric glandular lumen, especially around the parietal cells.

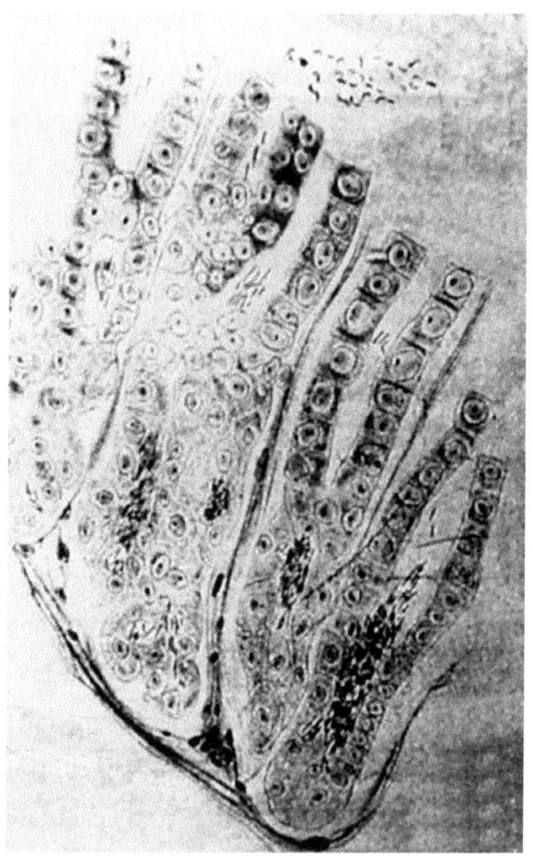

H. bizzozeronii, H. salomonis, which are contained in the broadly defined NHPH, are named after these pioneers.

3. From 1918 to 1982

Table 2 History of gastric mucosal spiral bacterium research from 1919 to 1975

1919	K. Kasai, R. Kobayashi	Salomonの報告を再現。猫からうさぎへの感染実験成功。サルバルサンによる除菌治療	NHPH
1920	R.K.S. Lim	猫の胃（胃体部、幽門部、噴門部）および十二指腸に螺旋菌を認めた	NHPH
1921	J.S. Edkins	Gastrin発見後、Helicobacter felis (?)の実験生理。猫の潰瘍との関係を報告。	NHPH
1924	J.M. Luck	胃粘膜にウレアーゼ活性発見	
1925	B. Hoffman	潰瘍症例胃組織をモルモットに投与し潰瘍形成、Bacilli Hoffmani の潰瘍形成性記載	
1930	B. Berg	部分迷走神経切離により潰瘍の二次感染阻止	
1939	J.L. Doenges	マカクザルと人で4種類のスピロヘータ感染, 壁細胞の傷害を認めた	Hp (?), NHPH
1940	A.S. Freedberg, L. Barron	人胃癌、胃潰瘍組織でスピロヘータ同定。Silver stainingを使う。病因との関係は不明。	Hp
1940	F.D. Gorham	潰瘍症形成における胃の酸嗜好性細菌の仮説。Bismuthで難治性潰瘍治療	Hp (?)
1946	M. Barber, R.H. Franklin	胃潰瘍感染説提唱	Hp (?)
1950	A.C. Ivy, M.I. Grossman, W.H. Bachrach	消化性潰瘍感染説を否定	
1953	H.L. Kornberg, R.E. Davies	胃内にウレアーゼを持った微生物	
1954	E.D. Palmer	剖検例でスピロヘータを否定、死後変化および口腔内常在細菌説	
1958	C.S. Lieber, A Lefevre	抗生剤投与で胃の尿素が減少し、脳症が改善	
1975	H.W. Steer	潰瘍における好中球遊走、菌を観察、分離、培養したが緑膿菌だった	P.aeruginosa

Shibasaburo Kitasato (1853-1931) was one of the earliest bacteriologists in Japan. He worked under Robert Koch and investigated tetanus and other bacterial infections. He was a founder of Kitasato University Nakamura and Matsui belong to now. In 1919, Shibasaburo Kitasato's youngest disciple, Rokuzo Kobayashi succeeded in infecting rabbits in addition to performing a follow-up test of Salomon's experiment using a spiral bacterium derived from a cat (9). Eradication therapy was also conducted using Salvarsan (arsphenamine), an antibacterial agent containing arsenic (Fig. 4).

Fig. 4 Spiral bacteria described by Kasai and Kobayashi.

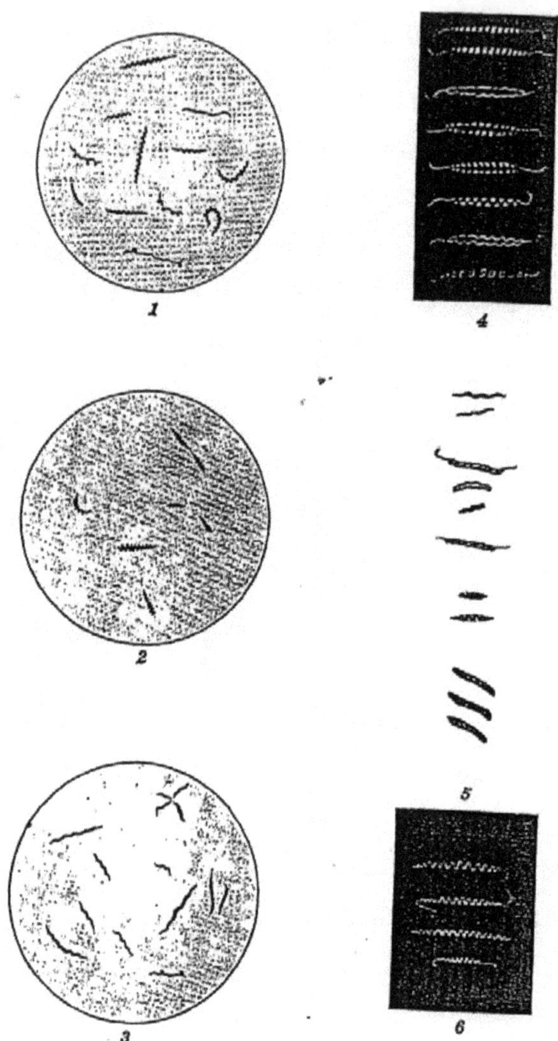

In 1939, Doenges reported four types of spiral bacteria from the examination of human autopsy cases (10), and he noted that a bacterium that was probably Hp occupied the main body of humans, and monkeys and other species. His report also described the presence of three species that were longer than Hp, similar to those reported in other animals.

In 1954, an examination of 1,180 autopsy cases by Eddy D Palmer of the Department of Gastroenterology at Walter Reed Army Hospital revealed that the spiral bacteria in the stomach were postmortem changes and were only indigenous bacteria only in the oral cavity (11). After that negative report, the theory of bacterial infection as the cause of gastroduodenal ulcer was ignored for 30 years. A factor that may have contributed to this is that at that time, physiological studies such as the discovery of gastrin related to gastric secretion were reported one after another. However, it is noteworthy that John Edkins, the discoverer of gastrin, subsequently conducted a study of cat ulcers and reported the involvement of a bacterium that appears to be NHPH, and most probably *Helicobacter felis* (12, 13). Gastric mucosal urease, which is now known to be related to *Helicobacter pylori*, was discovered by Murray Luck in 1924 (14). Conway reported in 1952 that urease activity was universally found in the stomach of mammals (15).

In addition, Kornberg *et al.* (16) and histochemical studies demonstrated that urease activity accumulated in the surface layer of the gastric mucosa, and they further showed the presence of microorganisms that decompose urease; they reported that the administration of antibiotics attenuated the urease activity. However, at that time, the relationships between urease-producing bacteria and gastric ulcer and gastric physiology were unclear; this may have been because that era was one of rapid progress in research on gastric acid secretion and its direct relation to gastric ulcer formation.

In 1975, Steer observed bacteria near epithelial cells in the gastric mucosal biopsy tissue of gastric ulcer patients. However, microaerobic culture was unsuccessful, and only *Pseudomonas aeruginosa* was identified; nevertheless, this was the first study to link bacterial infection and gastric ulcer (17), and it was a ground-breaking study that led to the work of Warren and Marshall. In 1979, Graham *et al.* reported epidemic gastritis with low acid, which was also related to Steer's report, suggesting a relationship among bacterial infection, gastritis, and gastric ulcer (18, 19). By that time, Robin Warren had already noticed the presence of bacteria in the stomach of patients with gastritis. Barry Marshall, a gastrointestinal intern, then attempted to culture this bacterium. An accidentally long-term culture was produced over Easter holiday ad was successful. Marshall reproduced the lesions by drinking the culture solution. The findings demonstrated by Warren and Marshall overturned many skeptical opinions and laid the foundation of our understanding of the significance of *Helicobacter pylori*. I think many of you are familiar with this story (20, 21). In the shadow of these discoveries, research on NHPH has slowly advanced.

Chapter 3 NHPH Nomenclature

NHPH was initially called Gastrospirillum hominis, but genetic analyses later revealed that it belongs to the genus Helicobacter. Its relationship within the genus Helicobacter was also clarified by the determination of the phylogenetic tree. Since several names for these bacteria had been used until recently, some confusion has arisen among reports.

1. From 1983 to 2005

Table 3 History of gastric mucosal spiral bacterium research from 1983 to 2005

Pre/Post	Year	First Author	Points	Hp/NHPH/others	Ref Number
Post-Hp	1983	B. Marshall	isolated and cultured H.pylori	Hp	20
	1985	B. Marshall, A. Morris	proved the infectivity by drinking the cultured bacteria (Koch postulate)	Hp	
	1987	J.C. Dent, et al	found strongly spiral bacteria in human gastritis tissue	NHPH	22
	1989	K. Heilman	found CLO (Campylobacter Like Organisms) in human biopsied tissue (in German)	NHPH	24
	1989	C.A.M. McNulty, et al	found strongly spiral bacteria in human type B gastrits, different from Hp	NHPH	23
	1990	E.N. Mendes, et al	found Gastrospirillum suis in pig stomach	NHPH	29
	1991	B.J. Paster	found Helicobacter felis in human gastric mucosa	NHPH	
	1993	J.V. Solnick. et al	proved Gastrospirillum hominis belong to Helicobacter species	NHPH	31
	1999	De Groote, et al.	named Gastrospirillum suis as Candidatus Helicobacter suis	NHPH	33
	1999	J.L. O'Rourke, et al.	postulated Helicobacter heilmannii type 1 (pig) and type 2 (cat, dog, other gastric NHPH)	NHPH	32
	2000	Morgner A, Stolte M, et al	reported H.heilmannii is more relevant to human MALT lymphoma than Hp	Hp, NHPH	74
	2005	J.R. Warren, B. Marshall	awarded the Nobel Prize in Physiology or Medicine		

Hp
NHPH

Immediately after the striking report by Warren and Marshall in 1983 (20), there were a series of reports of gastric spiral bacteria other than Hp from two groups; one from the UK led by J Dent and the other from Germany led by Konrad L Heilmann (22, 23). In April 1987, four years after the discovery of Hp, these groups observed spiral bacteria in the gastric mucosa of six patients with gastrointestinal symptoms; an Hp culturing method showed negative results. In a 1984 letter to Lancet, Clionda McNulty proposed that this bacterium be called *Gastrospirillum hominis Gen.nov., Sp.nov*. The bacterium was 3.5-7.5 μm long, 0.9 μm in diameter, and had up to 12 flagella on both poles. In 1987, Konrad Heilmann *et al.* made the first detailed pathological report (in German), followed by a report in English in 1991 (24, 25).

In that report, light and electron microscopic examinations were performed using endoscopically obtained specimens from patients with upper gastrointestinal symptoms, and this spiral bacterium was found in 39 patients (0.25%) of gastric mucosal tissue. Of these, 34 patients had chronic active gastritis; the remaining five had chronic gastritis. The symptoms of gastritis were improved by the administration of bismuth.

Much earlier in 1962, electron microscopic observations obtained by Weber *et al.* revealed the presence of spiral bacteria in the fundic gland mucosa of cats and dogs (26). Curry *et al.* described the existence of spiral bacteria in baboon stomach in 1987 (27). At the American Gastroenterological Association meeting in 1988, Dye, Marshall et al. proposed that a bacterium similar to the spiral bacterium of cats infects humans and causes gastritis (28). In 1990, Mendes *et al.* (29) identified a similar strain in the stomach of pigs and named it *Gastrospirillum suis* . This bacterium was renamed *Candidatus* H. suis in 1999 by DeGroote et al. (30).

Around the same time, Jay Solnick *et al.* infected mice with *Gastrospirillum hominis* from a patient and examined the 16S rRNA by PCR, and since the sequence of this bacterium resembled that of *H. felis*, it was classified in the genus Helicobacter (31). Solnick proposed the name *Helicobacter heilmannii. H.heilmannii*-positive cases were then accumulated and *H. suis* was classified as *Helicobacter heilmannii* type 1 based on 16S rRNA, and the other species were classified as type 2 (32-34). Type 2 species were also tentatively called *Candidatus* H. heilmannii (34).

In 2001, the presence of at least five types of *H. heilmannii*-like organisms (HHLO) in the human gastric mucosa was reported by Trebesius *et al.* (35). The name *H. heilmannii* was officially recognized in 2015 based on the success of the culture (36). In 2011, Freddy Haesebrouck *et al.* proposed the use of the term *Helicobacter heilmannii sensu lato* (*H. heilmannii sl*), for a Helicobacter bacteria other than *Helicobacter pylori* that inhabits the mammalian stomach (37). They also proposed that the term *sensu stricto (H. heilmannii ss)* to be used for species of *Helicobacter heilmannii.* 'non-*Helicobacter pylori* Helicobacter (NHPH)' is also used to indicate bacteria belonging to genus

Helicobacter other than *H. pylori* (38), divided into the gastric type and the non-gastric or enterohepatic type.

2. Summary of names

Table 4 summarizes the various names of genus Helicobacter that have been used to date. *Gastrospirillum hominis* and *Helicobacter heilmannii* were initially considered to refer to almost the same bacterium, but further research revealed more than one type, and as species, *Helicobacter suis, Helicobacter felis, Helicobacter bizzozeronii, Helicobacter salomonis, Helicobacter baculiformis, Helicobacter heilmannii sensu stricto, Helicobacter ailurogastricus*, and more are included.

Table 4 Various names of Helicobacter genus bacteria centered on NHPH

Helicobacter	gastric/enterohepatic	Hp/HHLO	gastric, non-gastric	type 1/2	Helicobacter heilmannii sensu lato	Species
Helicobacter Genus	gastric Helicobacter	Hp				*Helicobacter pylori*
		HHLO	gastric NHPH	*Helicobacter heilmannii type 1*	*Helicobacter heilmannii sensu lato*	*Helicobacter suis*
				Helicobacter heilmannii type 2		*Helicobacter felis*
						Helicobacter bizzozeronii
						Helicobacter salomonis
						Helicobacter heilmannii sensu stricto
						Helicobacter ailurogastricus
						Helicobacter cynogastricus
						Helicobacter baculiformis
						etc
	enterohepatic Helicobacter		non-gastric NHPH			*Helicobacter hepaticus*
						Helicobacter bilis
						etc
	others					*Helicobacter cinaedi*
						etc

In this book, for the sake of clarity, we use the generic term 'gastric NHPH' in the sense of HHLO, gastric NHPH and *H. heilmannii sensu lato*. When describing different characteristics of individual species, we will use each specific name, e.g. *H.heilmannii* and *H.suis*.

Chapter 4 Positive cases and positivity rates of NHPH

To date, over 800 cases NHPH-positive cases have been reported worldwide. Many of the reports of the positivity rate are limited to endoscopy examinees, and there is considerable variation, but conspicuously higher rate has been observed in East Asia compared to Western countries.

Table 5-1 Report of gastric NHPH cases from 1989 to 2000

Positive Case Number	Total Case Number	Year	First Author	Nation	Diseases: Gastritis	Nodular Gastritis	Gastric Ulcer	Duodenal Ulcer	Gastric MALT lymphoma	Gastric Cancer	Esophagitis	Others	Positive Rate	Bacterial Name	Definitive Diagnosis	Other Characteristics	Ref No.
1	1	1984	McNulty CA	UK	○ 1 case									spiral bacteria			39
1	2	1987	Dent JC	UK	○ 1 case									G. hominis	pathology		22
?		1988	Heilmann KL	Germany	?										pathology		40
6	8	1989	McNulty CA	UK	○ 6 case						○6 cases all negative		6/1300 (0.36%)	G. hominis	pathology		23
2	10	1989	Dye KR	USA	○ 2 cases									another spiral organism	pathology	first case 14 [illegible], second case two dogs	41
2	12	1990	Figura N	Italy								dyspepsia 2 cases	2/210 (0.95%)	spiral shaped bacteria	pathology	40yo male, 7yo female, 1/121 (0.83%) child case	42
4	16	1990	[illegible]	Germany	○ 4 cases									G. hominis	pathology		43
1	17	1990	Morris A	New Zealand	○ 1 case CAG								1/700 ([illegible]%)	tightly spiral shaped bacteria	pathology		44
4	21	1990	[illegible]	Italy	○ 4 cases								[illegible]%	G. hominis	pathology		45
2	23	1991	Borody TJ	Australia				○ 2 cases					DU 2/284 ([illegible]%)	G. hominis	pathology		46
1	24	1991	[illegible]	UK				○ 1 case (duodenal ulcer)						G. hominis	pathology	CLO test positive, duodenal mucosa positive	47
1	25	1991	[illegible]	Brazil										G. hominis	pathology	Hp mixed infection	48
1	26	1991	[illegible]	Italy	○ 1 case, CAG									G. hominis	pathology	[illegible]yo male, Hp mixed infection	49
39	65	1991	Heilmann KL	Germany	○39 cases antral active gastritis, body inactive gastritis									G. hominis	pathology		33
6	72	1992	Wegmann W	Switzerland	○ 6 cases									G. hominis	pathology		50
1	73	1993	[illegible]	Colombia	○ 1 case									G. hominis	pathology	2yo child	51
	73	1993	[illegible]	Brazil						○ 1 case				G. hominis	pathology	gastric cancer cases	52
2	76	1993	[illegible]	Switzerland	○ 2 cases								2/175 healthy cases (1.1%)	G. hominis	pathology		53
1	77	1994	[illegible]	USA	○ 1 case									G. hominis	pathology	[illegible]yo male using cats in experiment	54
1	78	1994	[illegible]	Japan	○ 1 case erosive gastritis									G. hominis	pathology	[illegible]yo male, medication success	55
1	77	1995	Morgner A	Germany						○ 1 case				H. heilmannii	pathology	50yo female, undifferentiated gastric cancer with mild gastritis	56
4	81	1995	[illegible]	Canada	○ 4 cases								4/912 (0.44%)	H. heilmannii	pathology		57
1	82	1996	[illegible]	USA			○ 1 case							G. hominis	pathology	14yo male gastric ulcer CAG, first north American child case	58
1	83	1996	Yang H	China						○ 1 case				H. heilmannii	pathology	[illegible]yo male, [illegible] CAG	59
1	84	1995	[illegible]	Japan	○ 1 case [illegible]									G. hominis	pathology	50yo female	60
14	98	1995	Debongnie JC	Belgium			○ 14 cases							H. heilmannii	smear cytology	14 Hh gastric ulcer cases compared with gastric ulcers with Hp or NSAIDs	61
202	300	1997	Stolte M	Germany	○ 2[illegible] cases		○[illegible] cases coexistence		○[illegible] cases coexistence	○ 1 case coexistence				H. heilmannii	pathology	compared with Hp gastritis	62
1	301	1997	Goddard AF	UK				○ 1 case						H. heilmannii	pathology	[illegible]yo male medication success with secondary regimen with TC	63
1	302	1997	[illegible]	Japan	○ 1 case erosive gastritis									G. hominis	pathology	[illegible]yo male	64
1	303	1997	[illegible]	Italy					○ 1 case	○ 1 case coexistence				H. heilmannii	pathology	gastric cancer and MALT lymphoma	65
20	323	1998	[illegible]	China	○ mild gastritis								20/[illegible] positive in Southern China general population	H. heilmannii	smear cytology, pathology		66
14	337	1998	[illegible]	Thailand	○ 14 cases, mild gastritis								14/267 ([illegible]%)	H. heilmannii	pathology		67
14	351	1999	[illegible]	Italy	○ 14 cases (0.01%)			○ [illegible] cases peptic ulcer		○ 1 case early carcinoma			0.01%	H. heilmannii	pathology	moderate gastritis, [illegible] Hp colonization, [illegible] gastritis	68
1	364	1999	[illegible]	Switzerland		○ 1 case						severe anemia		H. heilmannii	pathology	14yo male medication success with primary regimen	69
4	362	1999	[illegible]	USA			○ 1 case NSAIDs ulcer ([illegible]%)	○4 cases ([illegible]%)					4/1327 ([illegible]%)	H. heilmannii	pathology	positive with Hp immunohistochemical antibody	70
4	368	1999	[illegible]	Hungary	○ 1 case							○ 1 case [illegible]		H. heilmannii	pathology		71
3	369	1999	[illegible]	France	○ 1 case antral chronic gastritis	○ 2 cases							2/518 ([illegible]%)	H. heilmannii	pathology	3 child cases, Hp positivity [illegible]	72
1	372	1999	Yamamoto I	Japan	○ 1 case erosive gastritis									H. heilmannii	smear cytology, pathology	7yo male	73
5	377	2000	Morgner A	Germany					○ 5 cases					H. heilmannii	PCR	MALT lymphoma cases [illegible]	74

Table 5-2 Report of gastric NHPH cases from 2000 to 2020

Positive Case Number	Total Case Number	Year	First Author	Nation	Diseases: Gastritis	Nodular Gastritis	Gastric Ulcer	Duodenal Ulcer	Gastric MALT lymphoma	Gastric Cancer	Esophagitis	Others	Positive Rate	Bacterial Name	Definitive Diagnosis	Other Characteristics	Ref Number
33	406	2000	Svec A	Czechoslovakia	○ 33 cases								3%	H. heilmannii	pathology	big difference in prebalence, many cases in rural area	75
1	409	2000	Kamoshida T	Japan	○ 1 case antral gastritis									H. heilmannii	Pathology (Mckinlley)	38 yo male	76
8	417	2001	Ierardi E	Italy									8/7629 symptomatic cases (0.1%)	H. heilmannii	Pathology	2 cases doubly positive with Hp	77
1	418	2002	Yoshimura M	Japan	○ 1 case AGML									H. heilmannii	smear cytology, pathology	49yo female	78
1	419	2003	van Loon S	Holland	○ 1 case gastritis C1									H. heilmannii	PCR	8yo boy, identical DNA sequence of NHPH with two domestic cats	79
1	420	2003	Boyanova L	Bulgaria									1/321 (0.3%)	H. heilmannii	pathology	child case	80
1	421	2004	Wooten DC	USA	○ 1 case lymphocytic gastritis									H. heilmannii	pathology	19mo girl	81
5	426	2004	Sykora J	Czechoslovakia								dyspepsia 5 cases	5/580 (0.9%)	H. heilmannii	pathology	out of 585 child dyspepsia cases, 26.4% Hp, 0.9% Hh (5 cases)	82
15	441	2005	Okiyama Y	Japan	○ 11 cases chronic gastritis				○ 4 cases				15/4074 (0.37%) (consecutive endoscopy)	H. heilmannii	pathology	cross reaction with Hp antibody	83
1	442	2005	Sato S	Japan	○ 1 case mild chronic gastritis									H. heilmannii	pathology	years after eradication of Hp+duodenal ulcer, Hh+ mild	84
1	443	2005	Singhal AV	USA	○ 1 case mild gastritis									H. heilmannii	pathology	44yo male, cross reaction with Hp antibody	85
1	444	2006	Orel R	Slovenia	○ 1 case, acute phlegmonous gastritis, severe									H. heilmannii	pathology	13yo girl	86
1	445	2006	Oyamachi M	Japan	○ 1 case gastritis C1							Barrett Esophageal ca	coexistence with gastric polyp	H. heilmannii	pathology	RUT+	87
1	446	2007	Sislo K	Czechoslovakia	○ 1 case									H. heilmannii	pathology	57yo male, reinfection of Hh 3years after eradication, quadruple Tx, pet eradication treatment	88
2	448	2007	Quallo	USA	○ 2 cases									H. heilmannii	pathology	11yo boy, 2yo girl	89
10	458	2007	Joo M	South Korea	○ 10 cases								10/5888 (0.17%) chronic gastritis cases, 3281 Hp+ (56.9%)	H. heilmannii	pathology		90
2	460	2007	Boyanova L	Brasil	○ 2 cases erosive gastritis								0.3%/gastritis or ulcer patients	H.heilmannii	pathology	11 yo girl, 15 yo male, background: 77.8% Hp positive	91
1	461	2009	Matsumoto	Japan	○ 1 case chronic gastritis									H.heilmannii s.s	PCR		92
1	462	2010	Joffrimani BK	UK	○ 1 case									H.heilmannii	PCR	57yo female, cat keeper	93
22	484	2012	Iwanczak B	Poland		○ 17 cases	○ 2 cases MDG	○ 2 cases MDG				○ 3 cases normal mucosa	0.20%	H. heilmannii	pathology		94
1	485	2012	Ohtaka M	Japan					○ Vitiligo plasmacytoma					H. heilmannii	pathology	40yo female	95
1	486	2012	Okamura T	Japan					○ 1 case					H. heilmannii	pathology, PCR	46yo male	96
178	664	2014	Liu J	China	○ 11.87% /Hp positive cases	?							11.87% /Hp positive gastric disease patients	NHPH	PCR	bizzozeronii, heilmannii ss, salomonis	97
1	665	2014	Matsumoto T	Japan			○ 1 case multiple gastric ulcer (angle)							H.heilmannii s.s	PCR	82yo female	98
1	666	2015	Goji S	Japan		○1 case								H. suis	PCR	48yo female	99
2	668	2016	Shiratori S	Japan	○ 2 cases									NHPH	PCR	48yo and 54yo male	100
1	669	2016	Kobayashi M	Japan		○ 1case								H.suis	PCR	40yo female, resistant bacteria	101
19	688	2017	Øverby A	Japan		○ 1case	○ 1case	○ 3cases	○ 14cases					NHPH	PCR		102
9	697	2017	Tsukadaira T	Japan	○9 cases								gastric metaplasia (7/9)	NHPH	pathology, PCR		103
1	698	2018	Nakagawa S	Japan	○ 1 case									H. suis	PCR	36yo male	104
1	699	2019	Takigawa H	Japan		○ 4case								NHPH	PCR	H.suis alone, no heilmannii	105
4	703	2019	Suzuki S	Japan	○ 4 cases									NHPH	PCR	4 cases of NHPH positive gastritis, endoscopic characteristics	106
56	759	2020	Nakamura M	Japan	○ 38 cases	○ 6 cases	○ 8 cases MDG	○ 1case	○ 11 cases			Sjogren synd 1case		NHPH	PCR		107
60	819	2020	Shafaie S	Iran	○ 17 cases		○ 26 cases	○ 17 cases						NHPDH	PCR	H. bizzozeronii, salomonis, heilmannii s. felis	108
sum					644	35	57	33	44	8	5						
					gastritis	nodular gastritis	gastric ulcer	duodenal ulcer	gastric MALT lymphoma	gastric cancer	esophagitis	others	Positive Rate				

The NHPH positivity rate

More than 70 reports of gastric NHPH cases have accumulated as of 2020, and the number of individual cases is at least more than 800 at least (Table 5). However, positive rates reported in the general populations are extremely low, and most of the reports are based on the prevalence among endoscopy patients with gastrointestinal symptoms. This is probably because it is difficult to collect such data from general populations, and because the main focus has been on endoscopic biopsy tissue of patients with gastrointestinal disease. Thus, close attention must be paid to the survey target when viewing the data; otherwise, an overestimation is possible.

Even if we look at the cases of upper gastrointestinal diseases on the premise that the rate of NHPH positivity is likely to be high, it is 1% or less in Western Europe and Japan, and 0.5% or less in many cases in east Asian countries, especially China. Compared with the positive rate of Hp in a given target population at that time, it seems that the positive rate of gastric NHPH is about 1/20th to at most 1/5th of that of Hp among individuals with upper gastrointestinal tract symptoms in Asian countries. It is reasonable to expect that the NHPH positivity rate would be even lower in Western countries. Let's take a look at various diseases and their potential links with NHPH.

NHPH and disease

Initially, chronic gastritis accounted for most of the cases in which NHPH was identified, but many positive cases of gastric ulcer, duodenal ulcer and gastric MALT lymphoma were eventually identified. Other cases have included nodular gastritis, erosive gastritis, acute gastric mucosal lesions (AGMLs), duodenal erosion, acute gastrostomy, esophagitis, and gastric cancer. Regarding AGMLs, it is important to keep in mind that in Western countries, AGML is classified as a gastric ulcer, whereas in Japan it is often regarded as one of the forms of acute gastritis.

Relationships among NHPH, chronic gastritis, nodular gastritis and gastric cancer

Most of the reports of gastric NHPH-positive chronic gastritis are inactive or mild gastritis, and active gastritis is rarely observed. In addition, since most of the diagnoses before 2009 were based on pathological findings, there is a restriction that mixed infections with Hp were difficult to identify, and the misidentification of Hp cannot be denied as mentioned below.

Nodular gastritis was conventionally thought to be a change that occurred at the time of an initial infection with Hp, but the descriptions of nodular gastritis together with gastric NHPH started with the report of gastric NHPH-positive cases by Schultz-

Suchtung *et al.* in 1999 (69). The number of reports of since then, especially in Japan.

Nodular gastritis is attracting attention because it is related to gastric cancer, so I think many of you are familiar with it, but I would like to mention a few points. Nodular gastritis is a form of gastritis in which nodules and granular ridges are uniformly observed (like goosebumps on the skin) by upper gastrointestinal endoscopy. It was first reported by Takemoto *et al.* in 1962 (109). Its nature has been described as hyperplasia of the crypt epithelium and the formation of lymphoid follicles (110), but not all ridges are accompanied by with the formation of lymphoid follicles. In 1986, it was reported by Czinn *et al.* described nodular gastritis using the name of "nodular antral gastritis" as one of the characteristic endoscopic images of Hp infection in children (111). Konno *et al.*'s 1999 investigation revealed that 90% of children infected with Hp present with nodular gastritis (112). In recent years, cases of nodular gastritis together with gastric cancer have been reported by Kamada (113) and Sugimitsu *et al.* (114), and these patients are now regarded as being at high-risk for gastric cancer. Such cases were often found in women and were frequent in the body of the stomach, the macroscopic type has been 0-IIc type, and the histological type was undifferentiated.

The first example of a report on the gastric NHPH + nodular gastritis in Japan is the joint research report in 2010 by our research group and Professor Shinichi Nakamura's group at Tokyo Women's Medical University (115, 116). I happened to be with Professor Nakamura at an academic conference, and since we had observed that the histological findings of gastric nodular gastritis were similar to those of MALT lymphoma (which will be described later), we consulted Professor Nakamura about PCR testing of nodular gastritis cases and then examined ~100 cases of this disease; two NHPH-positive cases were detected. With written consent, biopsy tissue from these patients was orally administered to mice, and the lesion was reproduced in the mice 3 months later. The bacterium was registered in the DDBJ (DNA Data Bank of Japan) as *Candidatus* Helicobacter suis SNTW101, and is still maintained *in vivo* passages. Several analyses of the bacterium are in progress.

As mentioned above, the vast majority of nodular gastritis cases are positive for Hp, but the determination of which bacterium is the most likely to be associated with gastric cancer is an important issue to for future investigation (117).

Association between NHPH and gastric MALT lymphoma

It has been clear for a long time that gastric MALT lymphoma and Hp are strongly related, and as can be seen from the "Hematopoietic Tumor Treatment Guidelines 2013 Edition" edited by the Japanese Society of Hematology (Fig. 5), gastric MALT lymphoma is recognized as one of the indications for *Hp* eradication worldwide. It has also been known that even Hp negative cases can be improved by eradication therapy, and the involvement of another bacterium was presumed as one of the explanations for this; gastric NHPH is one of the candidate bacteria. In fact, such cases have been accumulated.

Fig. 5 Treatment of MALT lymphoma in accord with the Hematopoietic Tumor Treatment Guidelines-2013 Edition

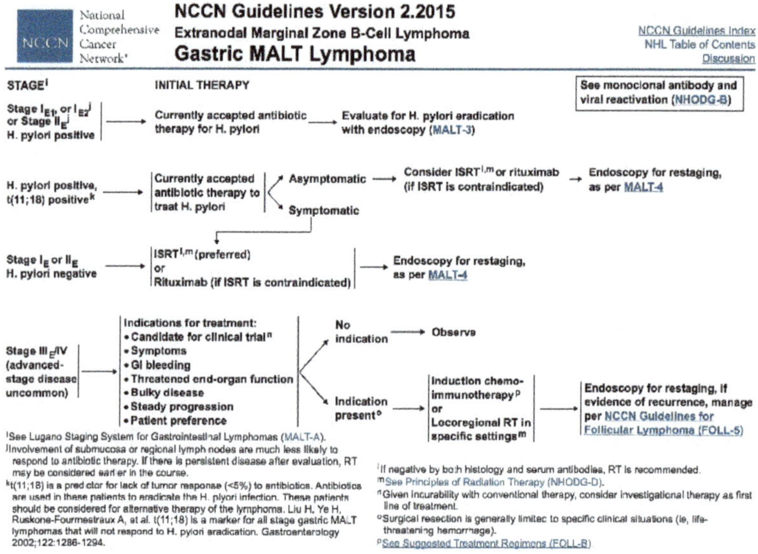

https://www2.tri-kobe.org/nccn/guideline/hematologic/nhl/english/mzl.pdf

Stolte *et al.* conducted a comparative study of 202 gastric NHPH-positive cases and 202 Hp-positive cases in 1997, and found that, unlike Hp, the localization of gastric NHPH is not diffuse, and gastritis, intestinal metaplasia, and lymphoma were mostly milder than Hp (61). However, seven cases of MALT lymphoma were included in the gastric NHPH-positive group, and thus the relationship between gastric NHPH and gastric MALT lymphoma is relevant. Stolte *et al.* therefore pointed out for the first time that it is necessary to consider the relationship between gastric NHPH and MALT lymphoma in detail.

Morgner *et al.* of the same research group later conducted an examination of gastric MALT lymphoma cases by histochemistry, specific immunoglobulin G-enzyme-bound immunoabsorption, and 16S rDNA nucleotide sequences, and they reported that five of the cases were gastric NHPH, not *Helicobacter pylori*, was positive. A study of cases from 1988 to 1998 identified gastric MALT lymphoma in 1,745 (0.66%) of 263,680 Hp-positive cases, and gastric NHPH in eight of 543 (1.47%) cases, indicating that compared to Hp, the gastric NHPH is more closely associated with gastric MALT lymphoma formation (73). In 2005, Okiyama *et al.* detected 15 gastric NHPH-positive cases (0.36%) among 4,074 consecutive biopsies, 11 of which exhibited chronic gastritis and four of which were gastric MALT lymphomas. (83). This appears to have been the first report of the relationship between gastric NHPH and gastric MALT lymphoma in Japan.

Øverby, one of our team members, compared the PCR positive rates of Hp and gastric NHPH using 282 cases of upper gastrointestinal tract disease and 64 controls obtained during the period 2005-2007 from five hospitals in Japan's Kanto region (102) (Table 6). His results demonstrated gastric NHPH-positive rates of 35% in gastric MALT lymphoma, 30% in duodenal ulcer and 5% in gastric ulcer. 21 cases of gastric MALT lymphoma had an Hp-positive rate of 52%. The analysis of the relationship between Hp and NHPH bacteria by Fisher's exact test revealed that gastric NHPH and Hp are independent factors.

Table 6 Relationship between gastric NHPH and *Helicobacter pylori*-positive rates and diseases in Japan's region from 2005 to 2007

Diseases	Number of Cases	NHPH-positive cases		Hp-positive cases	
		positive case number	%	positive case number	%
Gastric MALT Lymphoma	40	14	35%	21	53%
Gastric Carcinoid	1	0	0%	1	100%
GERD	16	0	0%	9	56%
Gastric Cancer	6	0	0%	6	100%
Nodular Gastritis	77	1	1%	57	74%
Duodenal Ulcer	10	3	30%	8	80%
Gastric Polyp	9	0	0%	3	33%
Superficial Gastritis	14	0	0%	5	36%
Atrophic Gastritis	88	0	0%	60	68%
Gastric Ulcer	21	1	5%	14	67%
Total Cases	282	19	7%	184	65%
Control Cases	64	0	0%	47	73%

Association between NHPH and gastric and duodenal ulcer

As of 2020, there are reports of at least 45 cases of gastric ulcer (Fig. 6) and 31 cases of duodenal ulcer that were positive for gastric NHPH. Many of these cases are were improved by the same treatment as that used for the primary eradication of Hp, but in rare cases, another drug was administered for secondary eradication (Table 7).

Table 7. Reports of gastric NHPH-positive cases of gastric ulcer and duodenal ulcer

Case Number	Year	First Author	Nation	Diseases: Gastritis	Nodular Gastritis	Gastric Ulcer	Duodenal Ulcer	MALT Lymphoma	Gastric Cancer	Esophagitis	Bacteria Name	Diagnosis	Ref Number
2	1991	Borody TJ	Australia				○2 cases				G.hominis	Pathology	46
1	1991	[illegible]	UK				○1 case duodenal erosion				G.hominis		47
1	1995	Akin OY	USA			○1 case					G.hominis	Pathology	56
202	1997	Stolte M	Germany	○202 cases		○8 cases		○7 cases	○1 case		H.heilmannii	Pathology	62
1	1997	Goddard AF	UK				○				H.heilmannii	Pathology	63
14	1999	[illegible]	Italy	○14 cases (0.01%)			○2 cases (past history)		○ Adenocarcinoma		H.heilmannii	Pathology	68
6	1999	Jhala D	USA			○2 cases NSAIDs Ulcer (0.71%)	○4 cases (0.42%)				H.heilmannii	Pathology	70
[illegible]	1999	[illegible]	Hungary	○1 case							H.heilmannii	Pathology	71
22	2012	[illegible]	Poland		○17 cases	○2cases Gastroduodenal Ulcer					H.heilmannii	Pathology	94
1	2014	[illegible]	Japan			○1case multiple gastric ulcer					[illegible]	PCR	98
19	2017	Øverby A	Japan		○1 case	○1 case	○3 cases	○[illegible]			NHPH	PCR	[illegible]
[illegible]	2020	Nakamura M	Japan	○[illegible] cases	○6 cases	○2cases Gastroduodenal Ulcer	○1 case	○[illegible]			NHPH	PCR	107
60	2020	[illegible]	Iran	○17 cases		○26 cases	○17 cases				NHPH	PCR	108
Sum				[illegible]	[illegible]	45	31	44	5	3			
				Gastritis	Nodular Gastritis	Gastric Ulcer	Duodenal Ulcer	MALT Lymphoma	Gastric Cancer	Esophagitis			

In the duodenal ulcer case reported by Goddard *et al.*, the patient's subjective symptoms did not improve after 1 week of treatment with omeprazole, clarithromycin, and metronidazole, and the result of a rapid urease test (which will be described later) remained positive. Treatment with omeprazole qd, de-Nol (bismuth subcitrate), tetracycline qid, metronidazole tid for 2 weeks was given and effective (63). There are also some cases related to AGML and duodenal erosion. In the reported cases of duodenal erosion, the gastric NHPH was found in the duodenal mucosa. Details of its eradication will be given in a later chapter.

A problem is that many people take nonsteroidal anti-inflammatory drugs (NSAIDs) these days, and it is thus necessary to clarify which factor is more relevant as the cause of a bacterial infection. Of course, in refractory cases, the exclusion of Crohn's disease and gastrinoma is essential.

Fig. 6 Endoscopic image of gastric NHPH-positive gastric ulcer case (98)

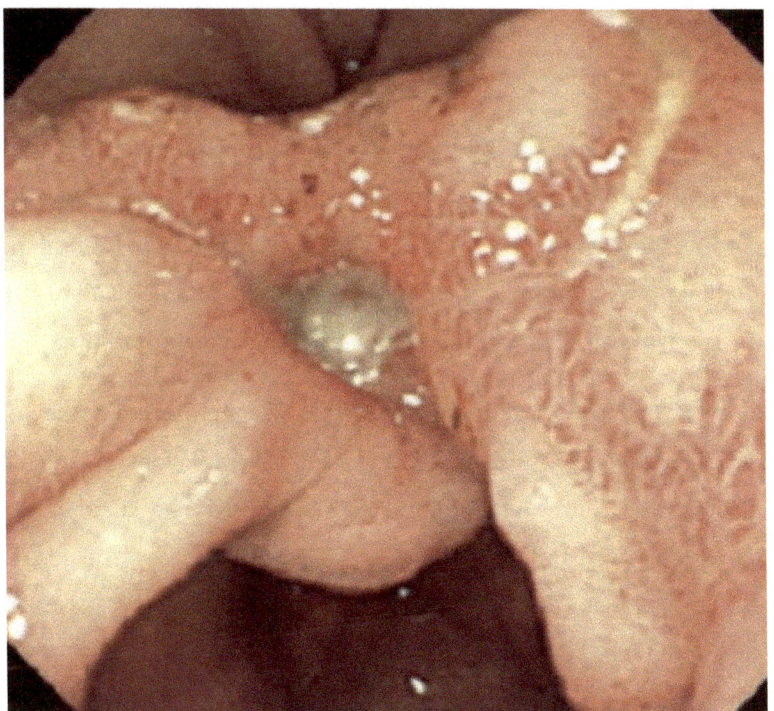

Association between NHPH and gastric cancer

Although there are sporadic reports on the relationship between NHPH and gastric cancer, there has been no cohesive analysis and no clear conclusions have been reached.

The first report (from Brazil by Nogueira *et al.*in 1993) described gastric cancer in a case of mixed infection with Hp and gastric NHPH (52). It was one of 40 gastric cancer cases, and the causal relationship of the gastric cancer is unknown due to the mixed infection.

The next report by Yang *et al.* in 1995 concerned a 49-year-old man with gastric cancer in the lesser curvature of the gastric antrum; gastric cancer (probably undifferentiated type from the findings) with chronic gastritis was diagnosed pathologically (59). The patient had a history of keeping dogs and cats in his home.

The same year, Morgner *et al.* reported a case of undifferentiated gastric cancer in a 50-year-old woman with an ulcer in the lower body of the stomach (56). The surrounding mucosa showed mild gastritis. In that report, one case of gastric cancer was identified in the authors' examination of 194 cases of gastric NHPH-positive gastritis. In the above-cited Yang *et al.* report, the rate was 1 in 51 cases, and there was concern that gastric NHPH might cause gastric cancer. Stolte *et al.* reported in 1997 that one of 202 patients with gastric NHPH-positive gastritis also had gastric cancer, and they described a relationship between single gastric NHPH infection and gastric cancer (62).

The same year, Goteri reported one case of collision cancer consisting of gastric NHPH-positive gastric MALT lymphoma and gastric cancer in a series of 12 cases of collision cancer (65).

Foschini *et al.* examined 14 patients who were positive for Hp in 1999 and they identified two cases of mixed infection with gastric NHPH, and one case with gastric cancer (67). All of the gastric NHPH-positive patients had mild to moderate gastritis.

After that study, for some reason, there have been few investigations of gastric cancer cases with gastric NHPH. Examinations of this type of case including the use of serodiagnoses, are a major task for future research, as is the relationship between NHPH and nodular gastritis as mentioned above.

Association between NHPH and acute phlegmonous gastritis

Acute phlegmonous gastritis is a non-specific purulent inflammatory disease that spreads mainly in the submucosa of the stomach wall, and Konjetzny has classified the causes of this gastritis into three groups; (*i*) the primary group, which has gastric origins (e.g., gastric ulcer, gastric cancer and other gastric diseases, foreign substances, and drugs); (*ii*) the secondary group from inflammation of nearby organs such as hematogenous infection or pancreatitis, cellulitis directly spreading from other infected foci (e.g., stomatitis and upper airway inflammation after tooth extraction), and primary disease caused by bacterial invasion from a damaged part of mucosa, and (iii) the third group with unknown origin (118). In the primary-group cases, the causative bacteria have been reported to be *Enterococcus faecalis, Enterobacter aerogenes, Klebsiella*, and others. In 2006, Orel *et al.* observed gastric NHPH in the gastric glandular cavity of patients with acute phlegmonous gastritis (86). However, this was only a morphological diagnosis, and the exact diagnoses were not obtained.

Association between NHPH and esophageal disease

McNulty *et al.* reported four patients with esophageal diseases in 1989, all of whom had gastric NHPH in chronic gastritis, but no bacteria have been reported in the esophagus (23), and a causal relationship with esophagitis formation is unknown. Oyauchi *et al.* reported a case of Barrett's esophageal cancer with mild gastric NHPH-positive gastritis (87). Testing for gastric NHPH in the esophagus in the case of Barrett’s esophageal cancer may help clarify the link, which is likely to be a coincidence.

Table 7 Suspected associations between diseases and gastric NHPH and Hp

Relation to Hp	Diseases	Evidence of Hp Eradication	Relation to NHPH
Indication of Hp Eradication	Chronic Gastritis	Effective, Improvement of Atrophy	Some Relation
	Nodular Gastritis	Effective	Strong Relation
	Gastric Ulcer	Effective, Suppression of Relapse, Complication	Some Reports
	Duodenal Ulcer	Effective, Suppression of Relapse, Complication	Some Reports
	Gastric Cancer	Decrease of Asynchronous Cancer	Some Reports, Still Unsettled
	Gastric MALT Lymphoma	Effective in More than Half cases	Strong Relation
	Hyperplastic Polyp	Reduction in 70% of the Cases	Some Reports
	Hp-related Dyspepsia	Effective, Different from FD	Some Reports
	GERD	Effective in Many Case, Some Exacerbation	Some Reports
	Idiopathic Thrombocytopenic Purpura	Effective in More than Half Cases	Unknown
	Iron Deficiency Anemia	Effective in Some Cases	Some Reports
Possible Relation to Hp Infection	Chronic Urticaria	Slightly Improve in Some Cases, Some Exacerbation	Unknown
	Cap polyposis	Effective in Some Cases, still Unsettled	Unknown
	DLBCL	Effective in Some Cases	Unknown
	Rectal MALT Lymphoma	Effective in Some Cases, still Unsettled	Some Reports, Still Unsettled
	Parkinson Syndrome	Effective in Relation to Levodopa Treatment	Some Reports
	Alzheimer Disease	Unsettled	Unknown
	Diabetes Mellitus	Unsettled	Unknown
Unknown	Follicular Lymphoma	Unknown	Some Reports, Still Unsettled
	Sjögren Syndrome	Unsettled	Some Reports, Still Unsettled
	Type A Gastritis	No Relation to Hp	Speculated
No Relation	Idiopathic Ulcer	No Relation to Hp	Speculated

Table 8 summarizes the relationship between Hp and various diseases based on the revised guidelines of the Helicobacter Society of Japan. There have been reports suggesting Hp's associations with various diseases other than those mentioned herein. Regarding gastric NHPH, there are still many diseases that are limited to single case reports, and future data collection is awaited. I will touch on the possible association of NHPH and some other diseases in a later chapter.

Chapter 5 Diagnostic methods for gastric NHPH

In the past, the diagnosis of gastric NHPH was mainly performed by pathological examination, but the PCR methods and other DNA-based methods are now the most reliable methods. In addition to the progress provided by whole-genome analyses, examinations using specific antibodies are also being attempted.

First, for comparison, the diagnostic methods approved by Japan's national health insurance system for Hp should be considered (Table 6). The methods used to diagnose Hp are shown in the table 9, considering the health insurance coverage in Japan. We added the corresponding information for gastric NHPH.

Table 9 Methods used for diagnose *Helicobacter pylori* and gastric NHPH.

Surface/Point	Method	Coverage by Japanese Health Insurance	Relation to NHPH
Point Diagnosis	Rapid Urease Test RUT, CLO)	○	△ negative to weakly positive
	Pathology (wirth IH)	○	○ possible overestimation
	Cluture	○	△ depend on facility
	PCR	×	◎ gold standard
Surface Diagnosis	Urea Breath Test	○	△ nagative to weakly positive
	Serum Antibody	○	? under investigation
	Urine Antibody	○	? under investigation
	Stool Antigen	○	? under investigation

In the case of Hp, one method can be selected for coverage by Japan's health insurance system. However, if the first test is negative, one more method can be used. It is also permitted to carry out one of the two specified combinations only for the first-time examination. The methods are classified into point and surface diagnostic methods.

Difficulty in diagnosing gastric NHPH

The reason why the diagnosis of gastric NHPH has not been made very frequently is that it is difficult to culture this bacterium even if its existence is suggested by microscopic examination, and as described later, the rapid urease test (RUT) used for Hp, the urea breath test (UBT), and tests for serum antibody, urinary antibody, and fecal antigen are all negative or weakly positive in gastric NHPH. It is thus likely that there is (at present) no way to obtain a definitive diagnosis other than the PCR method, under the pathological suspicion of the existence of gastric NHPH. We have summarized the case reports and diagnostic methods in Table 10.

Table 10 The relationship between case reports of gastric NHPH and diagnostic methods

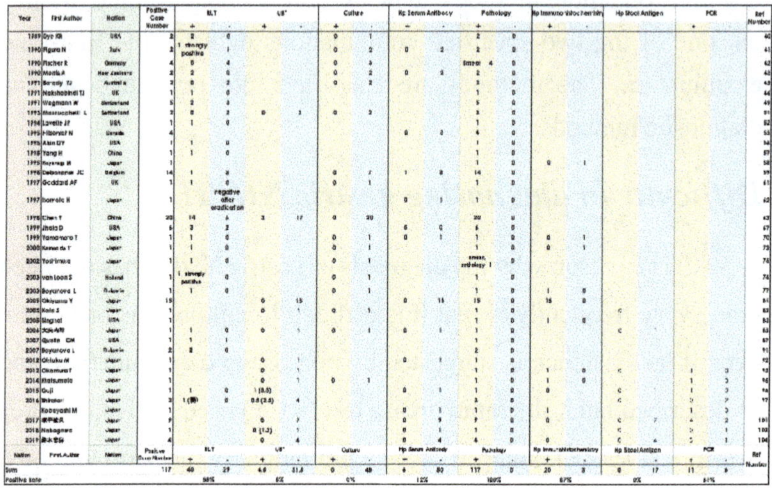

Year	First Author	Nation	Positive Case Number	RUT +	RUT -	UBT +	UBT -	Culture +	Culture -	Hp Serum Antibody +	Hp Serum Antibody -	Pathology +	Pathology -	Hp Immunohistochemistry +	Hp Immunohistochemistry -	Hp Stool Antigen +	Hp Stool Antigen -	PCR +	PCR -	Ref Number
1989	Dye KR	USA	2	2	0			0	1			2	0							40
1990	Figura N	Italy	2	1 strongly positive	1			0	2	0	2	2	0							41
1990	Fischer R	Germany	4	0	4			0	4			Smear 4	0							42
1990	Morris A	New Zealand	2	2	0			0	2	0	2	2	0							43
1991	Borody TJ	Australia	3	0	2			0	2			3	0							45
1991	Nakshabendi IJ	UK	1	1	0							1	0							46
1991	Wegmann W	Switzerland	5	2	3							5	0							49
1993	Mazzucchelli L	Switzerland	2	0	2	0	2	0	2			2	0							51
1994	Lavelle JP	USA	1	1	0							1	0							52
1995	Hilzenrat N	Canada	4							0	4	4	0							55
1995	Akin OY	USA	1	1	0							1	0							56
1995	Yang H	China	1	1	0							1	0							57
1995	Hayanagi M	Japan	1									1	0	0	1					58
1996	Debongnie JC	Belgium	14	1	8			0	7	1	8	14	0							59
1997	Goddard AF	UK	1	1	0			0	1			1	0							61
1997	Isomoto H	Japan	1		negative after eradication					0	1	1	0							62
1998	Chen T	China	20	14	6	3	17	0	20			20	0							63
1999	Jhala D	USA	6	3	2					6	0	6	0							67
1999	Yamamoto T	Japan	1	1	0			0	1	0	1	1	0	0	1					70
2000	Kaneda T	Japan	1	1	0			0	1			1	0	0	1					73
2002	Yoshimura	Japan	1	1	0			0	1			smear, pathology 1	0							74
2003	van Loon S	Holland	1	1 strongly positive	0			0	1			1	0							76
2003	Boyanova L	Bulgaria	1	1	0			0	1			1	0	1	0					77
2005	Okiyama Y	Japan	15			0	15			0	15	15	0	15	0					81
2005	Kato S	Japan	1			0	1	0	1			1	0			0				82
2005	Singhal	USA	1									1	0	1	0					83
2006	[illegible]	Japan	1	1	0	0	1	0	1	0	1	1	0			0				85
2007	Qualia CM	USA	1	1	1							1	0							87
2007	Boyanova L	Bulgaria	2	2	0							2	0							91
2012	Ohtsuka M	Japan	1			0	1			0	1	1	0							92
2012	Okamura T	Japan	1			0	1					1	0	1	0	0		1	0	93
2014	Matsumoto	Japan	1			0	1	0	1			1	0	1	0			1	0	95
2015	Goji	Japan	1	1	0	1 (8.5)				0	1	1	0	0		0		1	0	96
2016	Shiratori	Japan	3	1	0	0.8 (2.5)	4					3	0			0		3	7	97
	Kobayashi M	Japan	1							0	1	1	0	1				1	0	
2017	[illegible]	Japan	9			0	9			0	9	9	0	0		0	7	4	2	101
2018	Nakagawa	Japan	1			0 (1.3)	1			0	1	1	0			0		0	1	102
2019	[illegible]	Japan	4			0	4			0	4	4	0	0		0	4	3	1	104
Nation	First Author	Nation	Positive Case Number	RUT +	RUT -	UBT +	UBT -	Culture +	Culture -	Hp Serum Antibody +	Hp Serum Antibody -	Pathology +	Pathology -	Hp Immunohistochemistry +	Hp Immunohistochemistry -	Hp Stool Antigen +	Hp Stool Antigen -	PCR +	PCR -	Ref Number
Sum			117	40	29	4.6	51.8	0	48	6	80	117	0	20	3	0	17	11	6	
Positive Rate				58%		8%		0%		12%		100%		87%		0%		61%		

About the rapid urease test

For Hp, the RUT is the most frequently used r test along with serodiagnosis. Since Hp is often diffusely and abundantly distributed in the mucous layer in the stomach, it can be easily detected by the RUT by taking a sample from both the fundic gland and antral gland area.

When the RUT has been is used for the diagnosis of gastric NHPH, the reports have been divided into positive and negative cases. Summarizing the positive rates obtained to date, the average is 58% as shown in table 9, which is far below the result of 90% or more in the case of Hp. Moreover, the RUT method is considered difficult to use for the diagnosis of gastric NHPH. Even if a RUT result is classified as positive, the reaction varies from weakly positive to strongly positive, but is mostly weakly positive. The cause is thought to be the patchy distribution of gastric NHPH and the small amount of bacteria compared to Hp. Gastric NHPH is generally thought to adapt to animals other than humans and when the mice are infected with this bacterium is richly distributed in the mucus layer in both the fundic and antral mucosa in comparison with Hp, which gradually decreases in Hp-infected mice. When the urease activity is examined using an infected animal sample in the same manner as that used for humans, it shows a strong positive result, indicating that the reaction is dependent on the amount of bacteria. Among the genes described below, it is also known that gastric NHPH has a gene for urease similar to Hp. The distribution of gastric NHPH in the human stomach is focal, and the urease reaction is quite different depending on the site; the optimal site for biopsy from the viewpoint of endoscopy is not clear. Dr. Katsuhiro Mabe and Dr. Mototsugu Kato of Hakodate national hospital (Hokkaido, Japan) have demonstrated that marble-like endoscopic findings are characteristic of gastric NHPH, and it is hoped that a biopsy method more suitable for diagnosis be developed in future studies.

The urea breath test

The urea breath test examines the same urease activity and contributes to a so-called surface diagnosis, which can evaluate the entire stomach and is evaluated numerically. This test is therefore considered to be the most reliable method for identifying Hp. However, our examination of the reports of gastric NHPH-infected cases indicates that only 8% were positive, and even the positive cases showed only slightly higher positivity than the cutoff value. We suspect that the positive rate is too low compared to the results provided by the RUT, but this point needs to be clarified by accumulating a greater number of cases.

The uses of serum and urinary antibody

Herein, our use of the terms 'serum antibody' and 'urinary antibody' indicates only antibodies against Hp, and antibodies with high specificity due to gastric NHPH, which is currently under study.

The ABC classification for Hp infection frequently used with the serum antibody, and it has come to be used in medical examinations for gastric health check in Japan. The diagnostic accuracy is 88-100% sensitivity and 50-100% specificity according to the Helicobacter Society of Japan guidelines. It has also become clear that even if Hp is successfully eradicated, the titer of this antibody does not immediately normalize. On the other hand, in a study using this antibody against gastric NHPH, 12% positive cases were reported, but all have been negative since 2000 (Table 9). This may be due to the increased specificity of the antibodies used.

The pathological diagnosis and immunohistochemistry methods

A pathological examination usually uses samples that have undergone permanent preservation, and in the case of Hp, a histological diagnosis (i.e., evaluation of the degree of inflammation, atrophy, intestinal metaplasia and histological diagnosis of the disease) can be combined with a pathological examination in addition to the visual observation of the bacterium'a presence; its presence; this is one of the advantages in the diagnosis.

According to the Helicobacter Society of Japan guidelines, it is desirable to use special staining such as Giemsa staining in combination with hematoxylin and eosin (H & E) staining. Immunostaining is (in this case) a method of staining cells with a monoclonal or polyclonal antibody against Hp. The immunostaining is useful when it is difficult to determine the bacterium by a non-specific staining method, such as when one is differentiating Hp from other bacteria, when the number of bacteria is small, or when the bacteria take a coccoid form. An individual's treatment with a proton pump inhibitor may cause Hp to change to a coccoid form, move to the deep part of the gastric pit, and/or invade the intracellular canaliculus of parietal cells (although we have some doubts about this description)(Nakamura, Frontiers in Pharmacology, in press).

Pathologically, gastric NHPH is often morphologically distinguishable from Hp, but the spotty distribution of the bacterium is an important concern; some cases could be diagnosed as negative. There is an additional problem with the morphology of the spiral bacteria that exhibit long spiral morphology being swept with a broom. This is because Hp can exhibit both the usual short-spiral morphology and a long-spiral morphology (Fig. 7) (119). It is one of the reasons why PCR is important as the final step in the diagnosis of gastric NHPH.

In examinations by immunohistochemistry, it is clear that among cases in which H&E staining suggests gastric NHPH, 87% positivity has been shown in immunohistochemistry using an antibody against Hp according to the Helicobacter Society of Japan guidelines. Although it has been reported that gastric NHPH are positive with the Hp antibody from Dako (Glostrup, Denmark) (98), it is highly possible that the result will differ depending on the type of antibody used and thus depending on the recognition site of the antibody; thus, when an antibody is used to help reach a diagnosis, it is of course necessary to examine the reaction using positive and negative controls. However, it has been pointed out from the beginning that gastric NHPH is a bacterium that is related to and cross-reactive with Hp.

Fig. 7 Changes in the morphology of Hp depending on culture conditions (119)

When Hp is cultured on a blood agar plate, it shows the characteristic short spiral morphology of Hp, but in broth, Hp takes the form of a long spiral bacterium similar to gastric NHPH.

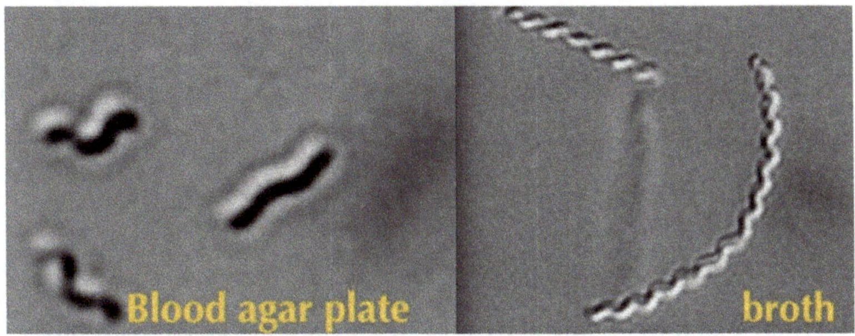

The fecal antigen test

The fecal antigen test detects antigens derived from Hp excreted from the stomach via the digestive tract. It is a method of directly detecting antigens, and the currently kits use monoclonal antibodies against Hp.

In this method, the antigenicity of Hp is described in the kits' package insert to be retained in the bacteria of the coccoid form bacteria, and the diagnostic accuracy is considered to be excellent, with a sensitivity of 96-100% and a specificity of 97- 100%.

In the package inserts of the fecal antigen test kits, gastric NHPH is said to be negative, and so far only negative cases have been reported. However, regarding the negativity, the statement states that the test was conducted using the ATCC (American Type Culture Collection) reference strain, but in many cases the authors' experience did not allow successful culture. Confirmation by case-based examination may be necessary to show its specificity.

Fig. 8 Results of rapid diagnosis of fecal antigen of the feces in the colon in gastric NHPH-infected mice

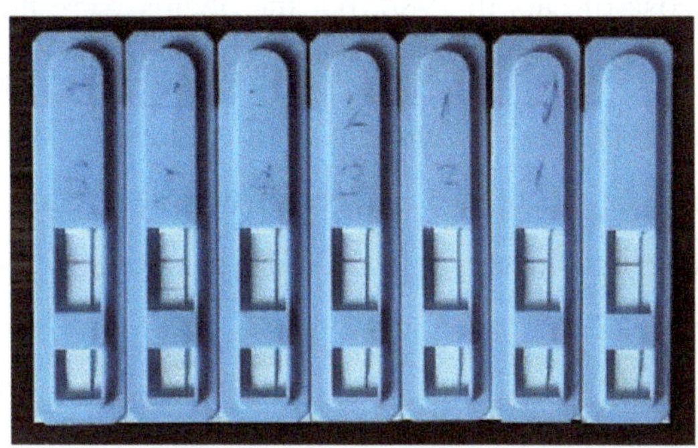

[table footnote] Since the samples were collected from the intestine, no contamination was considered, but positive cases were sometimes observed.

Culture of gastric NHPH

According to the guidelines, Hp grows under "slightly aerobic (5% oxygen, 15% carbon dioxide, 80% nitrogen) or 10% carbon dioxide conditions, but it takes 4 -7 days to culture. If round colonies ~ 2mm in diameter are observed, it is considered to be a colony of Hp. Gram staining is negative, and S-shaped spiral corkscrew movements can be observed with a phase-contrast microscope. The results of urease and catalase tests are positive.

Gastric NHPH is even more difficult to culture and has not been successful until recently.

Lee *et al.* reported culturing spiral bacteria from the antral gastric mucosa of cats in 1988, but the details were not provided. Two years earlier, Andersen *et al.* reported that they successfully cultured *Helicobacter heilmannii ss* in a medium similar to that used for Hp (121), but that bacterium was later confirmed to be another bacterium in the gastric NHPH bacterium, *Helicobacter bizzozeronii* (122).

Baele *et al.* reported successful cultivation of *Helicobacter suis* from the stomach of pigs in 2002 (123).

In 2011, the entire genome sequences of *Helicobacter suis* and *Helicobacter felis* were reported one after another (see the next chapter). The main points of this method are to soak the stomach cut in half in 1% HCl solution for 1 hour, add charcoal and HCl to the medium to make pH 5.0, and a microaerobic environment, and add 20% fetal calf serum (FCS) on the agar medium. Brucella broth was layered to prevent the medium from drying out (124). We also cultivated *Helicobacter heilmannii ss* from cats in collaboration with Bram Flahou *et al.* (Fig. 8-10) (125). Rimbara *et al.* reported a successful culture of *Helicobacter suis* from endoscopically obtained human biopsy tissue. (126) By applying this method, it is expected that the diversity of gastric NHPH and new bacterial species will be clarified in greater detail.

Fig. 9 Electron microscope image of cultured *Helicobacter heilmannii ss.* Fragments of flagella are also observed.

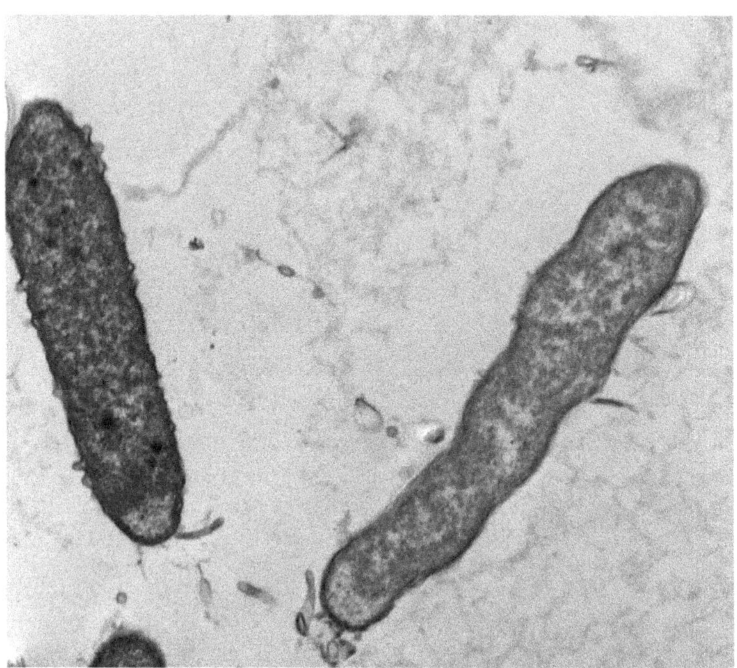

Figure 10 Cultured *Helicobacter heilmannii ss*

Cat-derived bacteria were donated by Dr. Bram Flahou, and Anders Øverby with Dr. Matsui cultured the bacteria. The image is from Time Lapse Vision (Shiki, Japan).

http://heilmannii.versus.jp/pg293.html

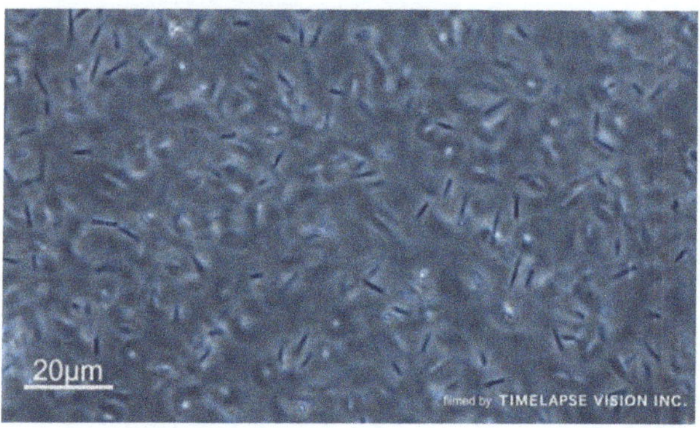

Figure 11 Still image of cultured *Helicobacter heilmannii ss.*

Flagella on both ends are observed.

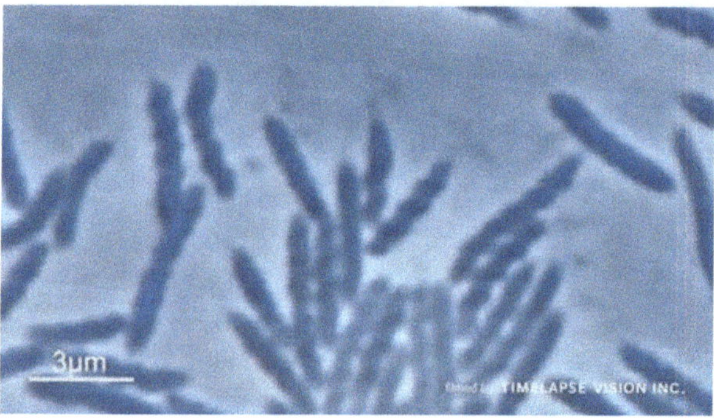

Chapter 6 Elucidation of the phylogenetic tree and genome of NHPH

The characteristics of the genome of gastric NHPH demonstrate that, like Hp, the sequence is highly diverse, it evolves in a region-specific manner, and there is a large amount of interspecies mixture. Various analyses continue to reveal inter-relationships.

As a new diagnostic method for gastric NHPH, in 2001 Trebesius *et al.* selected 84 of 543 cases of NHPH gastritis in Germany from 1989 to 1998, and they identified 5 types of gastric NHPH by fluorescent *in situ* hybridization (FISH) and 16S rDNA sequencing (127). Gastric NHPH has been found to infect humans, and most of these bacteria have been *Helicobacter suis*.

Fig. 12 Distribution of various gastric NHPH by the FISH method (125)

A: "*H. heilmannii*" type 1, B: "*H. heilmannii*" type 2, C: HHLO-4, D: HHLO-5 cells are stained yellow.

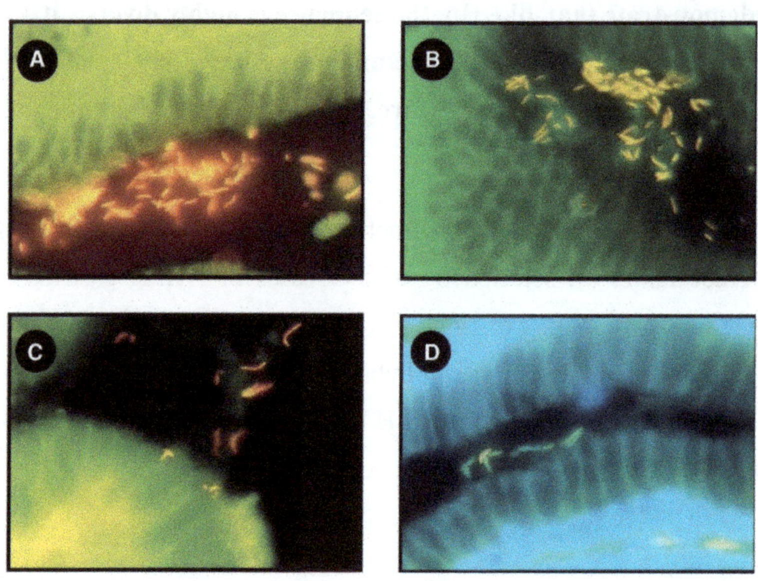

Chisholm *et al.* devised a new PCR system to detect gastric NHPH in biopsy tissue in 2003, 2.3% positivity among patients with dyspepsia in southeastern England, which is a significantly higher rate than previously reported (126). The next year, O'Rourke *et al.* created a phylogenetic tree of 26 strains of *Gastrospirillum hominis* 16S rRNA and urease genes obtained from humans and animals, of which 15 strains from humans, primates, and pigs were

"*Candidatus* Helicobacter suis", and the remaining 14 strains were classified as *H. felis, H. bizzozeronii, H. salomonis* and "*Candidatus* H. heilmannii" (127).

As mentioned in the previous chapter, Baele *et al.* reported the successful cultivation of *Helicobacter suis* in 2008, and in 2011, the total genome sequences of *Helicobacter suis* (128) and *Helicobacter felis* (129) were listed one after another. A comparison with Hp revealed that *H. suis* genome does not have the cytotoxicity-related protein (CagA), but has cag23 / E and cagX which comprise cagPAI. It was also reported that *Helicobacter suis* genome has almost the complete gene of the outer membrane proteins HpaA and HorB, which are considered to be the attachment factors of Hp, plus the type IV component system (ComB). It was revealed that there are genes homologous to Hp neutrophil-activating protein, γ-glutamyl transpeptidase (GGT), flavodoxin, and vacuolating cytotoxin A genes, which are related to the pathogenicity of Hp. In *H. felis* genome, Cag PAI and VacA were not found, but ComB, GGT, immunomodulator (NapA), collagenase and secretory serine protease (HtrA), which are attracting attention as virulence factors of Hp, were found.

The *H. felis* genome is characterized by a large number of chemotaxis sensors and restriction / modification systems. The entire genome sequences of *Helicobacter bizzozeronii* (130) isolated from the cases of severe gastritis and *Helicobacter heilmannii* (131) isolated from the gastric mucosa of kittens with severe gastritis were also reported.

Fig. 13 The phylogenetic tree based on the 16S rDNA base sequence of the genus Helicobacter

The strains in blue are the strains referred to as gastric NHPH.

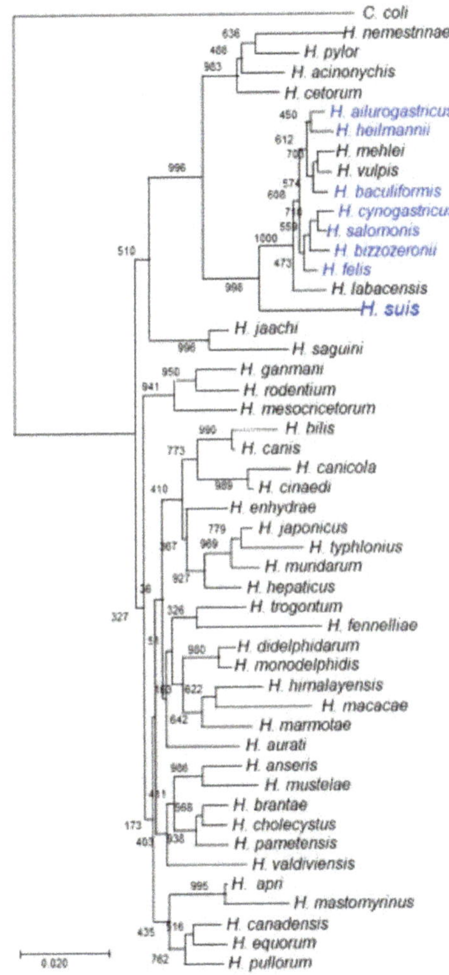

Figure 13 is a phylogenetic tree based on the 16S rRNA gene (16S rDNA) nucleotide sequence data-selected from the List of Prokaryotic Names with Standing in Nomenclature (http://www.bacterio.net/index.html) for 48 species of the genus Helicobacter that have been recognized as official names academically. obtained from NCBI

(http://www.ncbi.nlm.nih.gov/nucleotide). *Helicobacter apri* was proposed as a new strain in the International Journal of Systematic and Evolutionary Microbiology in April 11, 2016,but has a 16S rDNA base sequence of 1,099 bp, which is extremely short compared to those of other species.

Of the 16S rDNA (1,503 bp) of Hp, which is a representative species of the genus Helicobacter, 1360 bp (51 to 1,409) is common among 47 species other than *H. apri*, so we compared those parts. A multiple sequence comparison was performed with Clustal W (ver. 2.1, http://clustalw.ddbj.nig.ac.jp/index.php?lang=ja). The 16S rDNA of *Campylobacter coli* was used as an outgroup. Table 10 provides the list of 16S rDNA used in the phylogenetic tree shown in Figure 13. Table 11 lists the studies- we evaluated as sources of reference strains of Helicobacter spp.

The phylogenetic tree of 16S rRNA divides the Helicobacter species into two clusters. One contains in addition to Hp, *H. bizzozeronii, H. felis, H. heilmannii, H. mustelae, H. salomonis, H.*

suis and other gastric types that inhabit mainly the stomach; i .e., they are the gastric type NHPH (gNHPH)) ; *H. bilis, H. canis, H. cinaedi, H. fennelliae, H. hepaticus, H. pullorum, H. typhlonius*, and the others inhabit mainly the lower gastrointestinal tract below the cecum and bile liver system and belongs to the enterohepatic species (EHSs), which may also be detected in the genus Helicobacter.

Table 11 List of 16S rDNA nucleotide sequences used in the phylogenetic tree (Fig. 13)

Species	Type strain	16S rRNA accession no	bp
Helicobacter acinonychis corrig. Eaton et al. 1993	CCUG 29263	M88148	1485
Helicobacter ailurogastricus Joosten et al. 2017	ASB7	CDMG01000009	1502
Helicobacter anseris Fox et al. 2006	MIT 04-9362	DQ415545	1473
Helicobacter apri Zanoni et al. 2016	A19	KP120975	1099
Helicobacter aurati Patterson et al. 2002	MIT 97-5075c	AF297868	1455
Helicobacter baculiformis Baele et al. 2008	M50	EF070342	1455
Helicobacter bilis Fox et al. 1997	Hb1	U18766	1652
Helicobacter bizzozeronii Hänninen et al. 1996	CCUG 35545	Y09404	1421
Helicobacter brantae Fox et al. 2006	MIT 04-9366	DQ415546	1474
Helicobacter canadensis Fox et al. 2002	NLEP-16143	AF262037	1457
Helicobacter canicola Kawamura et al. 2016	PAGU 1410	LC102854	1595
Helicobacter canis Stanley et al. 1994	ATCC 51401	L13464	1473
Helicobacter cetorum Harper et al. 2006	MIT 99-5656	AF292378	1495
Helicobacter cholecystus Franklin et al. 1997	ATCC 700242	U46129	1472
Helicobacter cinaedi (Totten et al. 1988) Vandamme et al. 1991	CCUG 18818	AF348748	1473
Helicobacter cynogastricus Van den Bulck et al. 2006	JKM4	DQ004689	1462
Helicobacter didelphidarum Shen et al. 2020	MIT 17-337	MH726196	1504
Helicobacter enhydrae Shen et al. 2020	MIT 01-6242	CP016503	1501
Helicobacter equorum Moyaert et al. 2007	EqF1	DQ307735	1454
Helicobacter felis Paster et al. 1991	ATCC 49179	M57398	1474
Helicobacter fennelliae (Totten et al. 1988) Vandamme et al. 1991	CCUG 18820	AF348746	1833
Helicobacter ganmani Robertson et al. 2001	CCUG 43526	AF000221	1418
Helicobacter heilmannii Smet et al. 2012	ASB1	HM625820	1403
Helicobacter hepaticus Fox et al. 1994	Hh-2	AF302103	1470
Helicobacter himalayensis Hu et al. 2015	80(YS1)	KJ716794	1487
Helicobacter jaachi Shen et al. 2017	MIT 09-6949	KP701326	1459
Helicobacter japonicus corrig. Shen et al. 2017	MIT 01-6451	EF373963	1471
Helicobacter labacensis Gruntar et al. 2020	L9	MH854508	1498
Helicobacter macacae Fox et al. 2013	MIT 99-5501	AF333338	1654
Helicobacter marmotae Fox et al. 2006	MIT 98-6070	AF333341	1473
Helicobacter mastomyrinus Shen et al. 2006	MIT 97-5574	AY742307	1760
Helicobacter mehlei Gruntar et al. 2020	L15	MH854509	1498
Helicobacter mesocricetorum Simmons et al. 2000	MU 97-1514	AF072471	1420
Helicobacter monodelphidis Shen et al. 2020	MIT 15-1451	MH726195	1504
Helicobacter muridarum Lee et al. 1992	ST1	AF302104	1478
Helicobacter mustelae (Fox et al. 1988) Goodwin et al. 1989	ATCC 43772	Z25747	1481
Helicobacter nemestrinae Bronsdon et al. 1991	ATCC 49396	X67854	1463
Helicobacter pametensis Dewhirst et al. 1994	B9A Seymour	AF302105	1481
Helicobacter pullorum Stanley et al. 1995	ATCC 51801	FJ236465	1473
Helicobacter pylori (Marshall et al. 1985) Goodwin et al. 1989	ATCC 43504	M88157	1503
Helicobacter rodentium Shen et al. 1997	MIT 95-1707	U96296	1423
Helicobacter saguini Shen et al. 2017	MIT 97-6194-5	AF107494	1803
Helicobacter salomonis Jalava et al. 1997	Inkinen	U89351	1441
Helicobacter suis Baele et al. 2008	HS1	EF204589	1451
Helicobacter trogontum Mendes et al. 1996	LRB 8581	U65103	1422
Helicobacter typhlonius Franklin et al. 2002	MIT 97-6810	AF127912	1614
Helicobacter valdiviensis Collado et al. 2014	WBE14	KF549903	1383
Helicobacter vulpis Gruntar et al. 2020	L2	MH854505	1498
Campylobacter coli (Doyle 1948) Véron and Chatelain 1973	LMG 6440	AF372092	1341

Table 12 Sources and evaluation studies of reference strains of 48 Helicobacter species

Species	Source		Valid publication
Helicobacter acinonychis	cheetah	gastritis	Int J Syst Bacteiol 1993, 43: 99-106
Helicobacter ailurogastricus	feline	stomach	Int J Syst Evol Microbiol 2017, 67: 529-531
Helicobacter anseris	goose	feces	Int J Syst Evol Microbiol 2006, 56: 2025-2027
Helicobacter apri	wild boar	gastric mucosa, cecum	Int J Syst Evol Microbiol 2016, 66: 2876-2882
Helicobacter aurati	hamster	gastrointestinal tissues	Int J Syst Evol Microbiol 2002, 52: 3-4
Helicobacter baculiformis	feline	stomach mucosa	Int J Syst Evol Microbiol 2008, 58: 357-364
Helicobacter bilis	mice	bile, livers, intestines	Int J Syst Bacteiol 1997, 47: 601-602
Helicobacter bizzozeronii	canine	gastric tract	Int J Syst Bacteiol 1996, 46: 160-166
Helicobacter brantae	goose	feces	Int J Syst Evol Microbiol 2006, 56: 2025-2027
Helicobacter canadensis	human		Int J Syst Evol Microbiol 2002, 52: 3-4
Helicobacter canicola	canine	feces	Int J Syst Evol Microbiol 2016, 66: 4299-4305
Helicobacter canis	canine	feces	Int J Syst Bacteiol 1994, 44: 370-371
Helicobacter cetorum	dolphins, whales	stomach	Int J Syst Evol Microbiol 2006, 56: 2025-2027
Helicobacter cholecystus	hamster	gallbladder	Int J Syst Bacteiol 1997, 47: 601-602
Helicobacter cinaedi	human	rectal swabs	Int J Syst Bacteiol 1991, 41: 88-103
Helicobacter cynogastricus	canine	gastric mucosa	Int J Syst Evol Microbiol 2006, 56: 1559-1564
Helicobacter didelphidarum	opossum	cloacal prolapses	Int J Syst Evol Microbiol 2020
Helicobacter enhydrae	sea otter	stomach	Dis Aquat Organ 2017, 123:1-11
Helicobacter equorum	horse	feces	Int J Syst Evol Microbiol 2007, 57: 213-218
Helicobacter felis	feline	gastric mucosa	Int J Syst Bacteiol 1991, 41: 31-38
Helicobacter fennelliae	human	rectal swabs	Int J Syst Bacteiol 1991, 41: 88-103
Helicobacter ganmani	mice	intestine	Int J Syst Evol Microbiol 2001, 51: 1881-1889
Helicobacter heilmannii	feline	gastric mucosa	Int J Syst Evol Microbiol 2012, 62: 299-306
Helicobacter hepaticus	mice	livers, intestinal mucosa	Int J Syst Bacteiol 1994, 44: 595
Helicobacter himalayensis	marmot	gastric mucosa	Int J Syst Evol Microbiol 2015, 65: 1719-1725
Helicobacter jaachi	marmoset	gastrointestinal tracts	Int J Syst Evol Microbiol 2017, 67: 2075-2078
Helicobacter japonicus	mice	stomach, intestines	Int J Syst Evol Microbiol 2017, 67: 2075-2078
Helicobacter labacensis	red fox	gastric mucosa	Int J Syst Evol Microbiol 2020, 70: 2395-2404
Helicobacter macacae	rhesus monkeys	feces	Int J Syst Evol Microbiol 2013, 63: 3931-3934
Helicobacter marmotae	woodchucks feline	livers intestines	Int J Syst Evol Microbiol 2006, 56: 2025-2027
Helicobacter mastomyrinus	rodents	liver, intestine	Int J Syst Evol Microbiol 2006, 56: 2025-2027
Helicobacter mehlei	red fox	gastric mucosa	Int J Syst Evol Microbiol 2020; 70: 2395-2404
Helicobacter mesocricetorum	hamster	feces	Int J Syst Evol Microbiol 2000, 50: 1699-1700
Helicobacter monodelphidis	opossum	gastrointestinal tract	Int J Syst Evol Microbiol 2020
Helicobacter muridarum	rodents	intestinal mucosa	Int J Syst Bacteiol 1992, 42: 27-36
Helicobacter mustelae	ferret	stomach	Int J Syst Bacteiol 1989, 39: 397-405
Helicobacter nemestrinae	macaque	stomach	Int J Syst Bacteiol 1991, 41: 148-153
Helicobacter pametensis	bird, swine	feces	Int J Syst Bacteiol 1994, 44: 553-560
Helicobacter pullorum	chicken, human	liver, duodenum, caecum	Int J Syst Bacteiol 1995, 45: 418-419
Helicobacter pylori	human	gastric mucosa	Int J Syst Bacteiol 1989, 39: 397-405
Helicobacter rodentium	mice	intestine	Int J Syst Bacteiol 1997, 47: 627-634
Helicobacter saguini	cotton-top tamarin	intestine, feces	Int J Syst Evol Microbiol 2017, 67: 2075-2078
Helicobacter salomonis	canine	gastric mucosa	Int J Syst Bacteiol 1997, 47: 975-982
Helicobacter suis	pig	stomach	Int J Syst Evol Microbiol 2008, 58: 1350-1358
Helicobacter trogontum	rat	intestine	Int J Syst Bacteiol 1996, 46: 916-921
Helicobacter typhlonius	mice	cecum	Int J Syst Evol Microbiol 2002, 52: 685-690
Helicobacter valdiviensis	bird	feces	Int J Syst Evol Microbiol 2014, 64: 1913-1919
Helicobacter vulpis	red foxes	gastric mucosa	Int J Syst Evol Microbiol 2020, 70: 2395-2404

Subsequent development

In 2014, our co-author Matsui reported new primes for the detection of human-derived *H. suis* (132), and in 2016, Joosten *et al.* reported the genome sequence of *H. ailurogastricus,* a cat-derived bacteria close to *H. heilmannii ss* (133). The Hp virulence factors IceA1, HrgA, and jhp0562-like glycosyltransferases that are present in the *H. heilmannii* sequence were not found in the low-pathogenic species, *H. ailurogastricus.*

Cao *et al.* compared the 75 known genomes of Hp with the 24 known genomes of 20 species of NHPH in 2016 (134). There were 1,173 common conserved protein families among the 75 Hp strains, and 673 were conserved among all 99 Helicobacter genomes. Most of the 155 genes in 79 regions that are conserved among Hp strains and unique to Hp that lacked in NHPH are pathogenic and adaptively associated ones, such as cag-pathogenic islands, babBs, sabBs, and ABC transporters, whereas there are still 54 genes which the biological functions remain unknown.

In 2020, the genome sequences of *H. monodelphidis* and *H. didelphidarum* (135), *H. himalayensis* (136), *H. labacensis* and *H. mehlei* and *H. vulpis* (137), and *H. suis* SNTW101c strains by Rimbara (138), additionally, *H. cinaedi* in 2018 (139), *H. enhydrae* in 2017 (140), and *H. japonicum* (141), *H. saguini* (142) and *H. typhlonius* (143) were all identified in 2016.

Table 12 shows the representative genomes of the genus Helicobacter and their details that have been announced to date. As of December 2020, 3,939 genome assembles had been reported. No genomic sequences have been reported for the seven species, *H. apri, H. canicola, H. mastomyrinus, H. mehlei, H. monodelphidis, H. nemestrinae,* and *H. vulpis*. Other bacterial species have not been completely analyzed, but the known genome sizes are 1.36 - 2.77 Mbp, GC% is 31.6% - 47.7%, the number of proteins is 1,298 - 2,332, the rRNA is 2 - 9, and the tRNA value is 36 - 41, and the number of genes identified is 1,349-2,601.

Table 13 Genome details of Helicobacter species

Species	Isolate	RefSeq (accession id)	Assemblly date	Level	Size (Mb)	GC%	Protein	rRNA	tRNA	Other RNA	Gene	Pseudo-gene	No. of assemblies
H. acinonychis	Sheeba[T]	NC_008229	2006/6/28	Complete	1.55	38.2	1,359	6	36	3	1,532	128	8
H. ailurogastricus	ASB7[T]	NZ_CDMG00000000	2015/8/17	Scaffold	1.58	47.6	1,467	3	37	3	1,554	44	6
H. anseris	2013ZJHSD2	NZ_JXTW00000000	2019/3/25	Scaffold	1.46	33.6	1,356	3	36	3	1,427	29	2
H. aurati	MIT 97-5075[T]	NZ_NXLW00000000	2018/8/7	Contig	1.97	35.3	1,770	3	36	3	1,844	32	2
H. baculiformis	427351_3	NZ_FZMF00000000	2018/1/30	Scaffold	1.67	45	1,549	3	38	2	1,665	73	1
H. bilis	Missouri	NZ_JRPH00000000	2019/5/22	Contig	2.46	34.9	2,076	3	36	3	2,328	210	12
H. bizzozeronii	CIII-1	NC_015674	2011/6/8	Complete	1.76	46	1,510	6	37	3	1,743	187	10
H. brantae	MIT 04-9366	NZ_NXLV00000000	2018/8/7	Contig	1.73	39.1	1,586	3	37	3	1,638	9	1
H. canadensis	MGYG-HGUT-01348	NZ_LR698957	2019/8/10	Complete	1.62	33.7	1,539	9	41	3	1,617	25	5
H. canis	NCTC 12740	NZ_KI669458	2013/12/13	Scaffold	1.93	45	1,769	7	39	3	1,864	46	4
H. cetorum	MIT 00-7128	NC_017737	2012/4/19	Complete	1.95	34.5	1,673	6	39	3	1,784	63	5
H. cholecystus	ERZ467480	NZ_FZNE00000000	2018/1/30	Scaffold	1.36	35.2	1,298	3	36	3	1,349	9	3
H. cinaedi	P01D0000	NZ_AP018676	2018/6/9	Complete	2.15	38.6	2,053	6	40	2	2,236	135	38
H. cynogastricus	329937_4	NZ_FZMQ00000000	2018/1/30	Scaffold	1.66	44.1	1,571	8	37	3	1,683	64	1
H. didelphidarum	MIT 17-337[T]	NZ_NXLQ00000000	2018/8/7	Contig	2.59	31.6	2,212	3	36	3	2,400	146	1
H. enhydrae	MIT 01-6242[T]	NZ_CP016503	2017/4/17	Complete	1.59		1,492	2	38	3	1,553	14	1
H. equorum	MIT 12-6600	NZ_NXLT00000000	2018/8/7	Contig	1.75	37.7	1,650	3	37	3	1,757	64	2
H. felis	JKM3	NZ_FZKW00000000	2018/1/30	Scaffold	1.65	44.6	1,562	3	37	3	1,659	54	23
H. fennelliae	NCTC13101	NZ_UGID01000001	2018/8/1	Contig	2.16	37.9	2,030	6	39	3	2,174	96	4
H. ganmani	MIT 99-5101	NZ_NXLS00000000	2018/8/7	Contig	1.82	36.7	1,786	3	37	3	1,869	40	1
H. heilmannii	ASB1[T]	NZ_CDMK00000000	2015/8/17	Scaffold	1.64	47.7	1,495	3	37	3	1,625	88	8
H. hepaticus	ATCC 51449	NC_004917	2003/6/26	Complete	1.8	35.9	1,762	3	38	2	1,848	43	1
H. himalayensis	YS1[T]	NZ_CP014991	2016/3/30	Complete	1.83	39.9	1,664	6	39	3	1,769	57	1
H. jaachi	MIT 09-6949[T]	NZ_JRPR00000000	2019/5/22	Contig	1.9	41	1,786	7	39	3	1,877	42	1
H. japonicus	MIT 01-6451[T]	NZ_JRMQ00000000	2019/5/22	Contig	1.95	35.7	1,842	3	38	2	1,971	86	1
*H. labacensis**	1.9[T]	NZ_QXQQ00000000*	2020/2/29	Shotgun	1.73		1,582	3*	37	2	1,787	159	
H. macacae	MIT 99-5501	NZ_KI669454	2013/12/13	Scaffold	2.37	40.6	2,004	6	39	3	2,086	34	2
H. marmotae	MIT 98-6070	NZ_NXLR00000000	2018/8/7	Contig	1.96	39.6	1,835	3	38	2	1,938	60	2
H. mesocricetorum	87012_3	NZ_FZPJ00000000	2018/1/30	Scaffold	1.83	34	1,785	3	37	3	1,878	50	1
H. muridarum	NCTC12714[T]	NZ_UGJE00000000	2018/8/1	Contig	2.26	32.6	1,863	6	38	3	1,993	83	5
H. mustelae	NCTC12198[T]	NZ_LS483446	2018/6/17	Complete	1.58	42.5	1,373	6	39	2	1,448	28	3
H. pametensis	95149_6	NZ_FZPI00000000	2018/1/30	Scaffold	1.42	40.1	1,349	3	37	3	1,397	5	4
H. pullorum	NCTC13156	NZ_UGJF01000001	2018/7/31	Contig	1.79	34.4	1,702	6	39	3	1,780	30	24
H. pylori	Puno135	NC_017379	2011/8/26	Complete	1.65	39	1,465	6	36	3	1,564	54	1697
H. rodentium	ATCC 700285[T]	NZ_JHWC00000000	2014/4/8	Contig	1.81	37	1,858	4	37	3	1,953	51	1
H. saguini	15-1458 (F3)	NZ_QBIV00000000	2019/12/28	Contig	2.75	34.8	2,332	6	38	3	2,507	129	5
H. salomonis	56878_6	NZ_FZMA00000000	2018/1/30	Contig	1.58	46	1,443	3	37	2	1,539	54	5
H. suis	HSMmR02019b	NZ_CABIKE000000000	2020/2/10	Contig	1.65	40.1	1,557	5	39	3	1,669	65	33
H. trogontum	50960_6	NZ_FZNG00000000	2018/1/30	Scaffold	2.77	33	2,229	6	38	1	2,601	327	5
H. typhlonius	MIT 97-6810	NZ_LN907858	2015/11/20	Complete	1.92	38.9	1,792	6	38	2	1,916	78	5
H. valdiviensis	WBE14	NZ_NBIU00000000	2018/6/18	Contig	2.18	31.8	2,040	3	37	3	2,156	73	1

Helicobacter species have a small bacterial genome of about 2 Mbps. Bacteria that live in the stomach (e.g., Hp) or in the small intestine (e.g., *Lactobacillus reuteri*) have a relatively small genome. Perhaps the location in a nutrient-rich environment limits the number of genes involved in the biosynthetic system (144).

In 2018, Mannion *et al.* compared the 17 strains of gastric NHPH and 45 strains of EHS for a total of 110 genomes (145). The genome sizes of EHSs are larger than those of gastric NHPHs and corresponds to various metabolisms. A comparison of the genomes of gastric NHPH, EHS and *Campylobacter jejuni* (a close relative species) revealed 19,024 orthologs, of which 1,008 were common (145). The gastric NHPH-specific ortholog is 2,708 and the EHS-specific is 14,102. Compared to EHS, gastric NHPH are enriched in methyl-receptive chemotaxis proteins and two-component signaling proteins. Perhaps the high number of chemotactic genes in gastric NHPH are beneficial in responding to environmental stimuli of nutrients close to gastric epithelial cells at acidic pH levels. EHSs do not have the ability to colonize in similar mucosa and cannot utilize monosaccharides such as glucose, but they rapidly metabolize amino acids and organic acids to incorporate pyruvate and diaethyl into the citric acid cycle.

Since urease is essential for bacteria living in the stomach, all gastric NHPHs carry the urease gene and some EHS strains do too. The exception is *H. enhydrae*, which was isolated from the stomach of sea otter but lacks the urease gene. The urease of EHS may be useful for the production of ammonia for nitrogen assimilation rather than the neutralization of acid in the small intestine (pH ~ 6.1) and liver (pH ~ 7.4). Urease-positive EHSs (*H. hepaticus, H. bilis,* etc.), unlike urease-negative EHSs (*H. cinaedi* and *H. rodentium*), cause cholesterol gallstones and hepatobiliary inflammation in mice (146) and precipitate calcium *in vitro*. (147).

Both gastric NHPH and EHS species involve various virulence factors, and Mannion *et al.* summarized them based on the results of genome analysis (Table 13) (146). It can be seen in the table that virulence factors have evolved according to the environment as have growth essential factors and lipopolysaccharide (LPS) with an O antigen structure.

Table 14 Helicobacter virulence factors (146)

Gastric NHPH	Shared	EHS
Flagellar sheath adhesin (*hpaA*)	Alkyl hydroperoxide reductase (*ahpC*)	Cytolethal distending toxin (*cdtABC*)
Outer Membrane Proteins (OMPs)	Flagella	Cj1419c/cj1420c-like methyltransferase for capsule biosynthesis/transport
alpA/hopC	Fibronectin domain-containing lipoprotein (*flpA*)	Cj1421c/cj1422c-like sugar transferases for capsule biosynthesis/transport
alpB/hopB	γ-glutamyltranspepetidase (*ggt*)	HHGI1 pathogenicity island containing T6SS and secreted effectors hemolysin coregulated protein (Hcp), valine glycin-repeat (VgrG) protein)
babA/hopS	Heptose-1,7-bisphosphate (HBP)	Iron-regulated outermembrane virulence (*irgA*)
babB/hopT	Lipopolysaccharide (LPS)	N-linked protein glycosyltransferase
homB	Neutrophil activating protein (*napA*) hemolysin corrson	Vacuolating cytotoxin precursor
hopZ	Peptidyl-prolyl cis-trans isomerase (*ppiD*)	
horB	Plasminogen-binding protein (*pgbB*)	
oipA/hopH	Serine protease high temperature requirement A, (*htrA*)	
sabA/hopP	Urease (*ureA, ureB, ureI, ureE, ureF, ureG, ureH*)	
sabB/hopO		
Toxin-like OMP		
TNFαinducing protein (Tip-α)		
Vacuolating cytotoxin (VacA)		
Cagpathogenicity island*		

*Only H pylori

Evolution of Helicobacter spp.

In 2017, Flahou *et al.* clarified that non-human primates transmitted gastric NHPH to pigs between 100,000 and 15,000 years ago, followed by sporadic transmissions to humans. It was revealed that gastric NHPH has a different evolutionary pathway from Hp (148). De Witte *et al.* showed that the gastric NHPH infection in pigs was a host jump from rhesus macaques rather than cynomolgus macaques among primates (149). Berlamont *et al.* of the same research group isolated 15 strains of *H. suis* from rhesus monkeys and 20 strains from pigs to examine antimicrobial resistance (150): two porcine-derived strains are fluoroquinolone-resistant, one porcine-derived strain is tetracycline-resistant, one porcine-derived strain and two monkey-derived strains are lincomycin-resistant, and one monkey-derived strain is spectinomycin-resistant. The fluoroquinolone resistance came from single nucleotide polymorphisms (SNPs) of gyrA gene mutations. The tetracycline and spectinomycin resistance were mutations in the ribosomal protein. Compared to the monkey-derived strains, the porcine-derived strains tended to have higher minimum inhibitory concentrations (MICs) values for ampicillin, tetracycline, and doxycycline, and SNPs were observed in penicillin-binding protein and ribosomal protein genes. We must be cautious about the use of antibacterial agents in livestock.

An analysis of the Helicobacter gene by Smet *et al.* in 2018 revealed that recombination had occurred between species (151). In their comparison of genomes of 108 gastric NHPHs and 54 EHSs, a high frequency of interspecies recombination was observed between *H. heilmannii* and *H. bizzozeronii*, which are the species most frequently isolated from cats and dogs. Recombination was also observed between Hp, *H. acinonychis* (derived from cats) and *H. cetorum* (derived from marine mammals) and the recombination of these two species do not share the same host, gastric NHPH was indicated to be an ancestor. These findings demonstrate that gastric NHPH evolved in parallel from the bacterial species separately from Hp. At the same time, it appears that Hp had a host jump from animals to humans before acclimatizing to humans. By determining the era in which this occurred, in the case of dogs and cats, it became possible to estimate the relationship with the time of these animals' domestication to some extent. The relationship between gastric NHPH and animals is addressed in a later chapter.

Chapter 7 Bacterial eradication

Bacterial eradication is clinically important and in most of the existing clinical reports, regimen used for *Hp* eradication were effective: there are few reports of resistant bacteria. There are also cases of interest in which different treatments were used for reasons such as drug allergies.

1. Standard therapy for Hp eradication in Japan

The standard Hp eradication therapy in Japan is a triple therapy consisting of proton pump inhibitor (PPI) or potassium ion-competitive acid blocker (P-CAB) + amoxicillin (AMPC) + clarithromycin (CAM) for 7 days as the primary eradication regimen. As a secondary therapy (when necessary), metronidazole (MNZ) is used instead of clarithromycin for 7 days. Although it is not covered by Japan's health insurance at the moment, a PPI + AMPC + sitafloxacin (STFX) is used as a tertiary eradication regimen (153).

2. Reports of the eradication of gastric NHPH

There are more than 30 reports of gastric NHPH eradication as of 2020, and a variety of treatments have been administered (Table 14). However, there is no simple and reliable method to confirm the successful eradication of gastric NHPH like the UBT for Hp. The judgment of eradication has thus varied, depending on factors such as symptoms, endoscopic findings, and pathological observation in combination with the results of immunohistochemistry. Many recent reports describe the use of PCR, but in the early reports, it was difficult to judge whether the bacteria were really eradicated. In addition to the conventional PCR using biopsy tissue, the determination of bacterial eradication by a PCR using gastric juice is promising from the viewpoint of surface diagnoses, and it is important to consider this method in the future.

Table 15-1 Summary of eradication methods (1989-2003)

Year	First Author	Nation	Disease (Number of the Cases)								Used Eradication Regimen	Other Features	Ref Number
			Gastritis	Nodular Gastritis	Gastric Ulcer	Duodenal Ulcer	Gastric MALT Lymphoma	Gastric Cancer	Esophagitis	Others			
1989	McNulty DAM	UK	○6						○9 no bacteria		Various kinds of treatment was tried i.e. H2 antagonists, bismuth, amoxicillin, metronidazole. [illegible] judged by symptom		23
1989	Dye KR	USA	○2								bismuth, amoxicillin, metronidazole, duration unclear. Successful eradication	first case keeping 14 cats, second case with 2 dogs	41
1990	Figura N	Italy								○dyspepsia 2	ranitidine, antacid, duration unclear, eradication judged by endoscopy; 2nd case no treatment	40 yo male, 73 yo female. Positive rate 1/191 (0.5%)	42
1990	Morris A	New Zealand	○CAG 2 cases										44
1991	Naqshbandi M	UK				○Duodenal Erosion					treated with colloidal bismuth subcitrate. Symptom improved	positive CLO test, found in duodenal mucosa	47
1991	Heilmann KL	Germany	○39								Eight cases were treated with bismuth subsalicylate. No symptom after 4 weeks		25
1993	Lopez JA	Colombia	○1								treated with antacid and cimetidine for 1 months. Decrease in bacterial amount	7 yo child	51
1994	Lavelle JP	USA	○1								treated with bismuth subsalicylate. Symptom improved	30 yo male. Used cats for experiment	54
1994	Tanaka M	Japan	○1 Erosive Gastritis								treated with minocycline, cimetidine for 1 month, successful eradication by pathology	68 yo male	58
1995	Hilzenrat N	Canada	○4								1 case recovered by antibiotics, 1 case no treatment but recovered. 1 case mixed infection with Hp		57
1997	Goddard AF	UK				○					unsuccessful after 1 week tx with omeprazole 20mg, erythromycin 250mg, metronidazole 400mg. After, omeprazole 40 mg 2x/D, De-Nol 120 mg 4x/D, tetracycline 500 mg 4x/D and metronidazole 400 mg 3x/D daily for 2 weeks, improved endoscopy and pathology after 10 weeks	42 yo male	63
1997	Isomoto H	Japan	○1 Corpus Gastritis								symptom improved by sucralfate, metoclopramide. After Ciprofloxacin 300mg 2W, improved endoscopy and no bacteria after 6 months	59 yo male	64
1998	Chen Y	China	○mild Gastritis								eradicated by old triple therapy of Hp		66
1998	[illegible]	Switzerland		○						○Severe Anemia	After treatment with omeprazole 20mg, clarithromycin 500mg, amoxicillin 1000mg 2x/D, 2w, improved endoscopically and no bacteria by pathology after 7 months	14 yo male	69
1999	Mention K	France	○1 Antral Chronic Gastritis	○							2 cases ranitidine, amoxicillin, metronidazole, one case recovered with no treatment	8, 6, 14 yo, anti-Hp positivity 46/518	72
2000	Morgner A	Germany					○5				omeprazole 40mg, amoxicillin 750mg 3x/D 2W. All cases recovered in endoscopy and pathology with no relapse	5 cases of MALT lymphoma	74
2000	Kamoshida T	Japan	○1 Antral Gastritis								lansoprazole 30mg/D, amoxicillin 1500mg/D, clarithromycin 400mg/D 2W. Improved in pathology and no bacteria found	58 yo male	76
2002	Yoshimura M	Japan	○1 AGML								treated with omeprazole, clarithromycin, metronidazole 2W. Improved in endoscopy and pathology	69 yo female, cat keeper	78
2003	van Loon S	Netherlands	○ 1								treated with omeprazole, amoxicillin, clarithromycin 10days, symptom and endoscopy improved	5 yo boy, 2 cats. Identical bacteria by gene analysis	79

Table 15-2 Summary of eradication methods (2004-2020)

Year	First Author	Nation	Disease (Number of the Cases)								Used Eradication Regimen	Other Features	Ref Number
			Gastritis	Nodular Gastritis	Gastric Ulcer	Duodenal Ulcer	Gastric MALT Lymphoma	Gastric Cancer	Esophagitis	Others			
2004	Sykora J	Czechoslovakia								lm	omeprazole 20 mg, amoxicillin 25mg/kg, metronidazole 20mg/kg 2x/D 4 wks 80% omeprazole, metro, clarithromycin 15mg/kg 2x/D, bismuth subsalicylate 262 mg 4x/D symptom improved	28/41% Hp, 0.3% Hh (heilmannii) in 580 dyspepsia child	62
2005	Okiyama Y	Japan	○ 11 Chronic Gastritis				○4				MALT lymphoma remission by eradication treatment	immunoreactivity with Hp antibody	65
2006	Kato S	Japan	○ 1 mild chronic gastritis								treatment with lansoprazole, clarithromycin, amoxicillin 7D. Eradication succeeded.	11yo boy, Hp- DU 3 years after DU treatment	64
2006	Cizel R	Slovenia	○ 1 acute phlegmonous gastritis								quadruple therapy (omeprazole, 20 mg b.i.d. ciprofloxacin, 250 mg b.i.d., clarithromycin, 250 mg b.i.d., metronidazole, 400 mg b.i.d.) for 2 weeks. Symptom recovered	13yo girl	66
2007	Sykora K	Czechoslovakia	○ 1								omeprazole 20mg, amoxicillin 25mg/kg, metronidazole 20mg/kg 2x/D 4 wks Reinfection after 3 years. Successful eradication by quadruple Tx(omep, amo, clar, metro)	11yo male Proliferation of bacteria in pets true	55
2007	[illegible]	USA	○ 2								?	11yo boy 7yo girl	60
2010	[illegible] DK	UK	○ 1								?	8yo female, cat keeper	63
2012	Iwanczak B	Poland		○ 17	○ 2 MDG	○ 2 MDG				3 normal gastric mucosa		4 cases of NHPH-positive gastritis	54
2012	Otsuka M	Japan					○ 1 plasmacytoma				7-day course of lansoprazole 30 mg twice a day, clarithromycin 200 mg twice a day and amoxicillin 750 mg twice a day. Remission after 7 months	40 yo female	85
2012	Okamura T	Japan					○ 1 plasmacytoma				eradication therapy (10 mg rabeprazole, 750 mg amoxicillin, 400 mg clarithromycin twice daily for 7 days) improved in endoscopy and no bacteria after 3 months	48yo male	56
2014	Matsumoto T	Japan			○ 1 multiple ulcer						treated with triple therapy (amoxicillin, clarithromycin, and lansoprazole) improved in endoscopy and no bacteria in pathology	67yo female	58
2015	Goji S	Japan		○1							7 day course of triple therapy consisting of esomeprazole, amoxicillin and clarithromycin, negative UBT after two months	48yo female	59
2016	Shiratori S	Japan	○ 2								After one week triple therapy with amoxicillin, clarithromycin and rabeprazole, UBT became negative.	48 yo male, 54 yo male	130
2016	Kobayashi M	Japan		○1							treated with lansoprazole (60 mg/d), amoxicillin (1500 mg/d), and metronidazole (500 mg/d) no change in endoscopy and bacteria present in pathology. Treated with vonoprazan (40 mg/d), amoxicillin (1500 mg/d), and sitafloxacin (200 mg/d) [illegible] bacteria and nodular change gradually disappeared	40yo female resistant bacteria	131
2017	[illegible] T	Japan	○9								after lansoprazole long-term treatment alone, bacteria disappeared		133
2018	Nakagawa S	Japan	○ 1								esomeprazole, metronidazole, and amoxicillin for 10 days, 3 months after, improved in endoscopy and pathology, bacteria disappeared by PCR	58yo male	134
2020	Nakamura M	Japan	○ 39	○ 6	○ 2	○ 1	○ 11			Sjogren synd 1	By PPI based triple therapy bacteria disappeared by PCR in 45 cases		137

Among case reports of Hp infection, the proportion of resistant bacteria was about 10% in the 2000s, but it was reported to be increased to 38% in 2013-4 from the Japanese Helicobacter Society guidelines. Only a few resistant strains of gastric NHPH have been reported, but in the 2016 paper by Kobayashi *et al.*, cases that required a tertiary eradication of Hp were described. In addition, because of the history of clarithromycin used in other diseases, there have been cases in which a secondary eradication regimen for NHPH that was equivalent to the secondary eradication of Hp was used (104).

It is necessary to clarify the proportions of resistant bacteria and to suppress the increases in their numbers by providing a more systematic selection of treatment methods and genetic analyses.

Chapter 8 Clinical reports from Japan

Since the 1994 report from Hirosaki University, case reports of gastric NHPH in Japan have accumulated, and they take various viewpoints. Researchers from Shinshu University reported a large number of continuous endoscopic cases, which provide valuable information about the infection rate. In a 2020 issue of *Helicobacter*, we reported the results of a nationwide survey sponsored by the Helicobacter Society of Japan.

In this chapter, although there are some overlapped cases, we discuss clinical cases of gastric NHPH reported in Japan. Table 15 summarizes the existing reports, but we speculate that some reports may have been missed.

Table 15 Case reports of gastric NHPH in Japan to date

Year	First Author	Gastritis	Nodular Gastritis	Gastric Ulcer	Duodenal Ulcer	MALT Lymphoma	Gastric Cancer	Esophagitis	Others	Bacteria	Diagnostic Method	Features	Ref Number
1994	Tanaka M (Aomori)	○ 1 case, erosive gastritis								*G. hominis*	Pathology	66 yo male, successful eradication	55
1995	Koyanagi M (Aomori)	○ 1case AGML								*G. hominis*	Pathology	50 yo female	60
1997	Isomoto H(Nagasaki)	○ 1case, corpus gastritis								*G. hominis*	Smear	59 yo male	64
1999	Yamamoto (Kagoshima)	○ erosive gastritis								*H. heilmannii*	Smear	71 yo male	73
2000	Kamoshida T (Ibaraki)	○ 1case, antral gastritis								*H. heilmannii*	Pathology (McMullen method)	58 yo male	76
2002	Yoshimura M (Nagasaki)	○ 1 case, AGML								*H. heilmannii*	Smear, Pathology	69 yo female	78
2005	Okiyama Y (Nagano)	○ 11 cases, chronic gastritis				○ 4cases				*H. heilmannii*	Pathology	cross immunoreactivity with Hp Ab	83
2008	Kato S (Miyagi)	○ 1 case, mild chronic gastritis								*H. heilmannii*	Pathology	11 yo boy, 3y after Hp eradication, mild gastritis	84
2006	Oyauchi M(Miyagi)	○ 1 case, gastritis C1							Barrett esophageal cance	*H. heilmannii*	Pathology	49 yo male, RUT+	87
2009	Matsumoto T(Nagano)	○ 1 case, chronic gastritis								*H.heilmannii ss*	PCR		92
2012	Ohtaka M (Yamanashi)					○ 1case plasmacytoma				*H. heilmannii*	Pathology	40 yo female successful eradication	95
2012	Okamura T (Nagano)					○ 1case				*H. heilmannii*	Pathology, PCR	46 yo male successful eradication	96
2014	Matsumoto T (Nagano)			○ 1 case multiple						*H.heilmannii ss*	PCR	62 yo female	98
2015	Goji S (Aichi)		○1 case							*H. suis*	PCR	48 yo female	99
2016	Shiratori S (Hokkaido)	○ 2 cases								NHPH	PCR	48 yo male, 54 yo male	100
2016	Kubuyani M (Nagano)		○ 1case							*H.suis*	PCR	40 yo female, resistant	101
2017	Øverby A (Tokyo)		○ 1case	○ 1 case	○ 3 cases	○ 14 cases				NHPH	PCR		102
2017	Tsukadaira T (Nagano)	○9 cases								NHPH	Pathology, PCR		103
2018	Nakagawa S(Aomori)	○ 1 case								*H. suis*	PCR	56 yo male	104
2019	Takigawa H (Hiroshima)		○ 4cases							NHPH	PCR	H.suis alone	105
2019	Suzuki S(Hyogo)	○ 4 cases								NHPH	PCR	gastritis 4 cases, endoscopic feature	106
2020	Nakamura M (Tokyo)	○ 35 cases	○ 6 cases	○ 2 cases	○ 1 case	○ 11 cases			Sjogren syndrome case	NHPH	PCR		107

The first positive case of gastric NHPH infection in Japan was reported by Tanaka *et al.* at Hirosaki University in 1994: a 66-year-old man with upper abdominal pain (55). Cimetidine alone subsided the inflammation but gastric NHPH remained observable in the mucosa. With minocycline and cimetidine administration, the bacteria diminished, and the gastric mucosa was normalized. Cases of AGML were reported by Koyanagi *et al.* from Hirosaki University (60) and Yoshimura *et al.* of Omura Municipal Hospital (78). Corpus gastritis cases were described by Isomoto *et al.* of Nagasaki University (64), and Kamoshida *et al.* of Hitachi General Hospital reported cases of antral gastritis (76).

In their investigation of 4,074 consecutive biopsies, Okiyama *et al.* of Shinshu University and Maruko Central Hospital found 15 gastric NHPH-positive cases, 11 of which were chronic gastritis and four of which were gastric MALT lymphoma (83).

In 2005, Kato *et al.*(Tohoku University) found that an 11-year-old boy with a duodenal ulcer was infected with gastric NHPH three years after a successful eradication of Hp, and the first-line eradication regimen for Hp was used to eradicate his gastric NHPH (84). Dr. Kato reported the details of this successful eradication, and this appears to be the first report of cases of pediatric gastric NHPH after Hp eradication.

In 2006, Oyauchi *et al.* (Tohoku University) described a gastric NHPH-positive case of Barrett esophageal cancer (87). It was reported that *H. suis* formed an ulcer in the anterior stomach of pigs, which histologically resembles the human esophagus. It is therefore important to determine whether gastric NHPHs are actually distributed in the esophagus in humans.

In 2014, our collaborator Shinichi Nakamura of Tokyo Women's Medical University identified two gastric NHPH positive cases among ~100 cases of nodular gastritis, which were generally attributed to the initial infection with Hp (116). In these cases, the RUT result was negative and the PCR test showed infection with NHPH alone (134). Many reports clarifying the relationship between gastric NHPH and nodular gastritis in Japan then followed, For example,

Goji and Sasaki (Aichi Medical University) reported in 2015 that one gastric NHPH-positive case identified by PCR was positive for urease by RUT and UBT, but were negative for Hp in serum antibody and fecal antigen tests (99). Shiratori and Mabe reported the endoscopic characteristics of gastric NHPH positive cases as a white-marble appearance in the infected antral mucosa in 2016 (100). In 2018, Nakagawa and Shimoyama (Hirosaki University) observed a red depressed lesion by endoscopy in a patient whose UBT, Hp fecal antigen, and Hp blood antibody were negative and PCR indicated a gastric NHPH-positive case (105). This bacterium was shown to be immunoreactive to the antibody against *Helicobacter suis* created by our group, suggesting the significance of this antibody for the diagnosis of *H. suis*.

In 2019, Suzuki and Terao of Kakogawa Central City Hospital identified four gastric NHPH-positive cases; 2 cases were *H. suis*-positive and the other two were positive for *H. heilmannii ss* by PCR (106). Endoscopically two cases showed edema, mild diffuse redness and mucosal swelling in the body of the stomach. The other two cases showed goose skin appearance in the antrum but no erosion, edema, or diffuse redness of the mucosa. No correlation between bacterial species and endoscopic findings have been established.

However, some features of endoscopic findings in gastric NHPH-positive cases have been gradually accumulated.

Results of joint research 2010-2013

In 2010, with the support of the Helicobacter Society of Japan, we started the "Nationwide Survey on Disease Formation Caused by *Helicobacter heilmannii, suis* (HHLO) Infection". We first surveyed hospitals in the Tokyo area from 2010 to 2013, and the results were summarized by Anders Øverby (102). The survey found subjects who were positive for gastric MALT lymphoma, gastric ulcer, duodenal ulcer and nodular gastritis. At that time, we were interested in gastric MALT lymphoma linked to NHPH, and these cases were intentionally gathered. We observed a strong relationship between gastric NHPH and MALT lymphoma. Regarding nodular gastritis, we have started joint research with Professor Shinichi Nakamura (Tokyo Women's Medical University) as mentioned above. Initially, only Hp-positive cases were found, but the 65th case was found to be the first Hp-negative case that was positive for gastric NHPH. After that report, additional Hp-negative cases were identified one after another, which triggered the next examination. In contrast, although we did not expect to find many cases of Hp-positive gastric and duodenal ulcers, several positive cases were identified (see Table 6 in Chapter 4 above).

Results of joint research 2013-2019

Next, in collaboration with gastroenterologists across Japan, we used PCR to examine the relationship between gastric NHPH and Hp in upper gastrointestinal tract diseases, and this time the analysis was focused on Hp-negative cases.

Fig 14 Joint research facilities and gastroenterologists across Japan

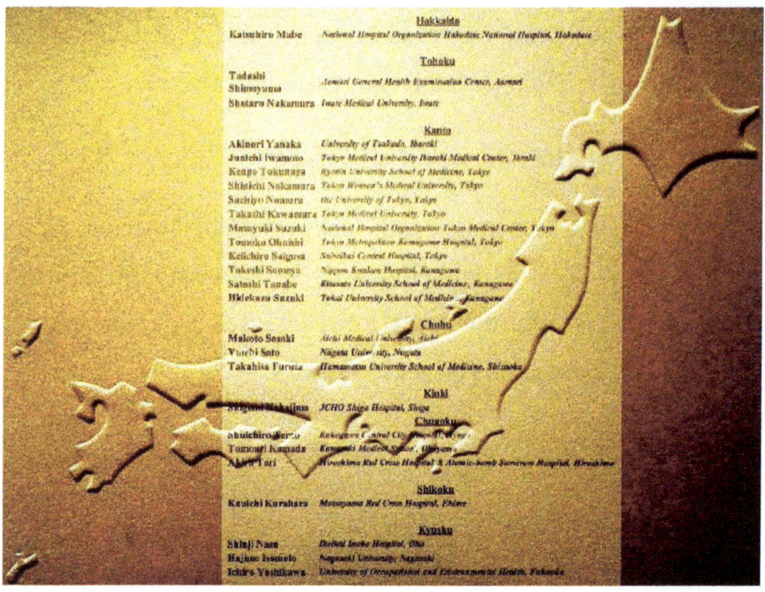

The analysis results demonstrated that among 236 non-eradicated Hp-negative cases by RUT, pathology and PCR, 20% of the cases were positive for gastric NHPH (Fig. 15). On the other hand, in the post-eradicated Hp-negative cases by RUT, pathology and PCR, about 10% were positive for gastric NHPH. Among the Hp-negative cases by RUT and pathology, 10% of the cases were found to be positive for Hp by PCR; this may be a limitation of the routinely used diagnostic method, although this matter is outside the scope of this book.

Fig. 15 Classification of target cases and summary of results

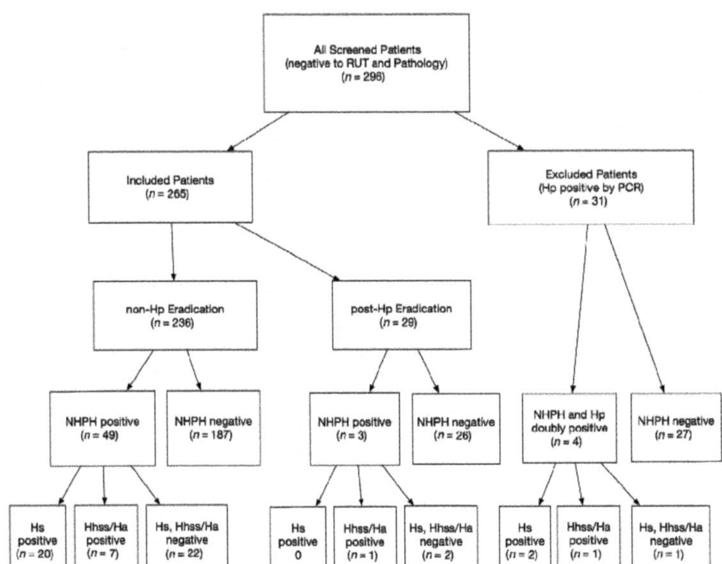

Next, looking at the relationship between NHPH and the disease, we observed that among gastric diseases, the proportion of gastric NHPH positivity was highest in the order of nodular gastritis, gastroduodenal ulcer, gastric MALT lymphoma, and chronic gastritis (Table 17). No gastric NHPH-positive cases were found at that time for duodenal follicular lymphoma or colon MALT lymphoma, which have been reported to be related to the gastric NHPH. On the contrary, in patients with Sjogren's syndrome, which is known to be associated with lymphoma, gastric NHPH was observed in gastric mucosa showing chronic gastritis. Whether this is coincidental or related seems to require a large number of case studies.

Table 17 Gastric NHPH-positive rate by disease

Diseases	Number of Cases	Positive Cases
total	**236**	**49 (20.8%)**
gastric MALT lymphoma	**46**	**11 (23.9%)**
chronic gastritis	**162**	**28 (17.3%)**
nodular gastritis	**15**	**6 (40.0%)**
gastroduodenal ulcer	**9**	**3 (33.3%)**
gastric cancer	**1**	**0**
polyp	**2**	**0**
SS	**1**	**1 (100%)**
duodenal follicular lymphoma*	4	0
colon MALT Lymphoma*	4	0

* not included in the total number

Looking at the associations between *H. suis* and *H. heilmannii ss* with diseases, none of the findings showed a significant association, and both species were shown to be involved in these diseases to the same extent (Table 18).

Table 18 Positive rates for *H. suis* and *H. heilmannii* ss by disease

Species	total	MALT lymphoma	Nodular Gastritis	Chronic Gastritis	Gastroduonal Ulcer	Sjögren Syndrome
total	49	11	6	28	3	1
H suis	20 (40.8%)	4	4	11	1	0
Hhss/Ha	7 (14.3%)	2	2	2	1	0
unidentified	22 (44.9%)	5	0	15	1	1

n.s.

Differences in the gastric NHPH-positive rate by geographic region

We had a hypothesis about regional differences in Japan based on the regional food consumption data. Figure 16 shows the results of a household survey by the Ministry of Internal Affairs and Communications. The difference between the consumption of a high amount of pork in eastern Japan and the high consumption of high amounts of beef in western Japan can be seen in the figures. Since the deviation values, and not the actual numbers are given, the difference may be enhanced, but in eastern Japan, pork is often added to curry rice, beef tends to be used (many Westerners are familiar with the high-quality Kobe beef from west Japan). There are several proposed explanations for how and why this regional difference in meat consumption developed, but it seems that cows were used in the western Japan for agriculture, and horses were used not only for agriculture but for military in eastern Japan; horse meat is difficult and unpleasant to eat, and pigs were thus raised for food.

We thus suspect that *H. suis*, whose natural host is pigs, is likely to be more prevalent Japan.

Figure 16 Differences in pork and beef consumption and pig and cattle breeding numbers by prefecture in Japan

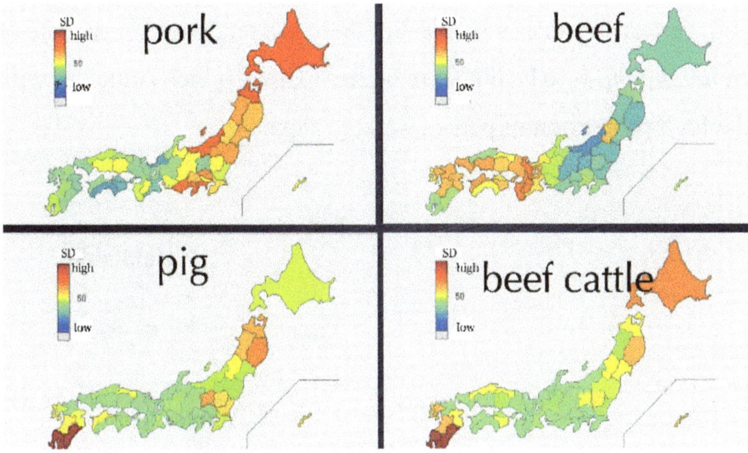

Looking at this national survey, it is clear that there are significant regional differences in the positive rate of gastric NHPH as a whole. In addition, *H. heilmannii ss* shows clear regional differences. This could be related to the higher rate of keeping pets in western Japan.

Figure 17 Regional positive rate of *H. heilmannii ss* and differences between eastern and western Japan

There is a significant bias in the regional distribution of species of gastric NHPH. In the data obtained to date, there is no significant difference in the distribution of the gastric NHPH between eastern and western Japan as a whole, but there is a tendency for the rate of *H. heilmannii ss* to be higher in western Japan, which coincides with the high proportion of pets in western Japan.

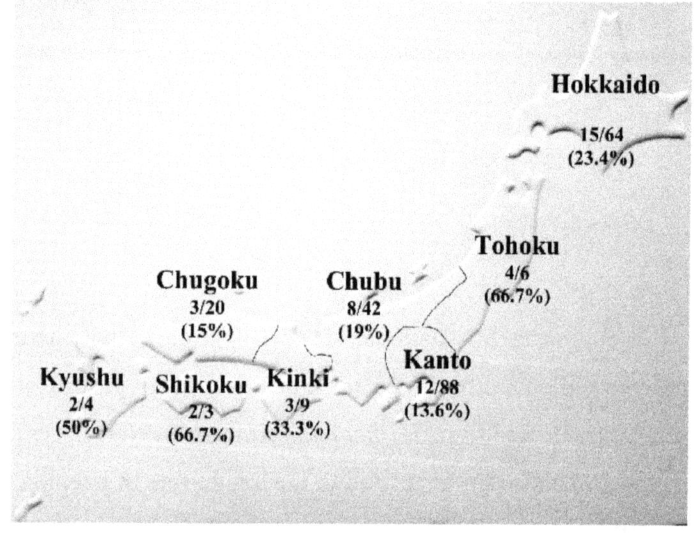

	All	East	West
all cases	236	200	36
all positive cases	49	39	10
Hs-positive cases	20	17 (44%)	3 (30%)
Hhss/Ha-positive cases	7	4 (10%)	3 (30%)
Undetermined cases	22	18 (46%)	4 (40%)

Chapter 9 The examination of gastric NHPH with experimental models, especially gastric MALT lymphoma

Gastric NHPH is not only morphologically different from Hp; its localization within the gastric mucosa also differs. We believe that at least some of the reported Hp in parietal cells may have been gastric NHPH. Several animal models have been used to investigate the relationship between gastric NHPH and MALT lymphoma, which was revealed in clinical cases.

Gastric ulcer, gastric MALT lymphoma, and gastric cancer can be induced by infecting various animal species with *H. heilmannii, H. suis*, and other gastric NHPH species (154). These species could probe a model of human disease and are useful to investigate the pathophysiology and treatment of gastric MALT lymphoma and other diseases.

Fig. 18 Diseases caused by Hp infection and the experimental model (154)

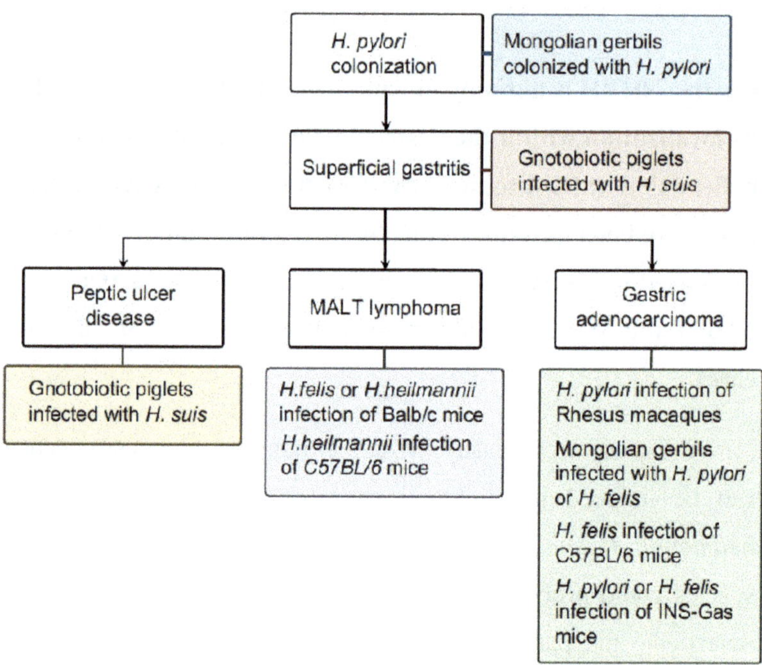

Animal models of MALT lymphoma are a good example.

Generally speaking, human gastric MALT lymphoma was thought to be caused mainly by Hp, but a series of reports including that by Stolte *et al.* in 2000 (74) revealed that some of these cases were caused by gastric NHPH.

Fig. 19 Distribution of cells in the gastric mucosa of *Helicobacter suis*-infected C57BL / 6 mice

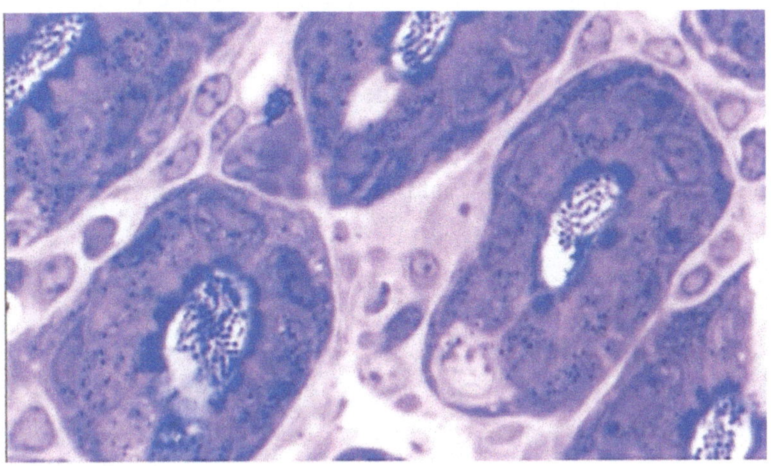

Gastric NHPHs that were stained with toluidinc blue are observed in the gastric glandular lumen of the infected mice, and one of them were detected in the parietal cells.

The concept of a MALT lymphoma experimental model

Various gastric NHPH species including *Helicobacter felis, H. heilmannii ss*, and *H. suis*, have been used for the examination of MALT lymphoma in animal experiments. Mainly BALB / c and C57BL / 6 mice were used in these studies. Experiments have been devised and selected from the perspective of whether the host animal can be infected with the bacterium of interest and whether the animal can form lesions with characteristics similar to those of human MALT lymphoma. However, compared to Hp, gastric NHPHs are difficult to culture for infection experiments, and doing so was not possible until recently, so in the form of animal-to-animal infection (*in vivo* passage culture). In the future, as the number of bacterial species that can be cultivated continues to increase, animal models could be achieved with a more effective infection method.

History of gastric MALT lymphoma animal experiments

Typical reports in which MALT lymphoma or lymph follicle formation has been reported since 1995, and their relation to eradication experiments using those systems are summarized in Table 19.

Table 19 History of animal models of gastric MALT lymphoma

Year	First Author	Species	Natural Host	Infected Animal	Period	Objective	Intervention	Results	Ref Number
1995	Enno	H.felis		SPF BALB/C mouse	22 months	Formation of MALT Lymphoma like lesion	—	after 22 months, lymph follicle 38%, LEL 25%, control 0%	138
1997	Erdman	H. mustelae	ferret	ferret (natural infection)	observation	Formation of MALT Lmphoma	—	low grade 50%, high grade 50%	139
1998	Enno	H. felis (ATCC49179)		BALB/c mouse	until 24 mo	Eradication Effect	Eradication by metronidazole, bismuth, tetracycline	improvement of lymph follicle formation and MALT lymphoma	140
1999	Dieterich	H. heilmannii	mouse	BALB/c mouse		Immunological Response by urease	Immunization by H. heilmannii Urease B and Hp urease	Inflammation attenuated, but gastric mucosal atrophy occured	141
2004	Park	H. suis	pig 6mo old	SPF ICR mouse	until 24 mo	Immunological Analysis	—	later than 8 wk lymphocyte, plasa cel infiltration, later than 64 wk lymph follicle formation, atypical mucosa	142
2004	O'Rourke	H. heilmannii	wild dog, rhesus macaque, macaque, mandrill monkey, bobcat, human	BALB/c mouse	24 mo	Pathological Analysis		later than 18 mo MALT lymphoma formation (25%)	143
2004	Fukui	H. pylori TN2GF4		thymectomized BALB/c mouse	until 12 mo	MALT Lymphoma Formation by Hp	—	80% MALT Lymphoma in thymectomized mouse, 0% control	144
2005	Helleman	H.suis	pig	SPF BALB/c mouse	administration after 2 weeks	Eradication Effect	Eradication by omeprazole and amoxicillin	decrease of fecal bacteria	145
2006	Helleman	H.suis	pig	SPF BALB/c mouse	immunization after 2 weeks	Immunological Response	nasal immunization with H. pylori, H. felis, followed by H. suis	urease activity decreased, no change in fecal bacteria,	146
2007	Nakamura	H.suis TKY	cynomolgus monkey, maintained in C3H mouse	SPF C57BL/6 mouse	until 18 mo	Time Course, Pathological Analysis	—	MALT lymphoma formation 50% (3 mo) 100% (6 mo later)	147
2007	Nishikawa	H.suis TKY	cynomolgus monkey, maintained in C3H mouse	SPF C57BL/6 mouse	until 18 mo	Relation to Microcirculation and VEGF	—	Increase in VEGF A, C immunoreactivity in Lymphoma. P cell apoptosis	148
2008	Nakamura	H.suis TKY	cynomolgus monkey, maintained in C3H mouse	SPF C57BL/6 mouse	until 18 mo	Relation to Flt-1 and COX-2	—	Increase in COX-II immunoreactivity in Lymphoma	149
2008	Park	H heilmannii	pig, maintained in C3H mouse	C57BL/6 mouse	until 18 mo	Immunological Analysis	—	Accumulation of CD45R+ cell, IFN-g, IL10 increase	150
2008	Matsui	H. suis TKY	cynomolgus monkey, maintained in C3H mouse	SPF C57BL/6 mouse	administration after 3 mo	Eradication Effect	Eradication	Not completely eradicated, but tumor size decrease	151
2010	Nakamura	H. suis TKY	cynomolgus monkey, maintained in C3H mouse	SPF C57BL/7 mouse	administration after 4 mo	Effect of VEGF Receptor antibody	VEGF receptor antibody	Tumor size decrease by Flt-1, 4 antibody	152
2010	Flahou	H. suis (HS1, 2, 3)	pig	mongolian gerbil, BALB/c mouse, C57BL/6 mouse	until 8 mo	Pathological Analysis	—	Parietal cell necrosis in mouse and gerbil, MALT lymphoma-like lesion in gerbil	153
2010	Suzuki	H. heilmannii (SH4)	human	SPF BALB/C mouse	until 83 weeks	Pathological Analysis	—	high endothelial cell with GlucNAc6STs	154
2010	Nobutani	H. suis TKY	cynomolgus monkey, maintained in C3H mouse	C57BL/6 mouse, Peyer's patch deficient mouse		Pathological and Immunological Analysis	—	MALT lymphoma formation without Peyer's patch	155
2017	Nakamura	H. suis TKY	cynomolgus monkey, maintained in C3H mouse	SPF BALB/C mouse	administration after 3 mo	Pathological Analysis	Effect of Substance P Antagonist	tumor suppression by substance P antagonist	156
2018	Kodama	H. suis TKY	cynomolgus monkey, maintained in C3H mouse	unilateral vagotomized SPF C57BL/6 mouse	administration after 4 mo	Pathological Analysis	Effect of Unilateral Truncal Vagotomy	MALT lymphoma enlarged in vagotomized side, interaction of substance P	157

Initially, Adrian Lee's group in Australia examined not only *H. felis* but also *H. heilmannii* and *H. suis* by using animals from Taronga Zoo in Sydney. These species were observed by transmission to humans (155-157, 160). Eradication was also studied, and the results have been applied to humans. Groups from Switzerland and Belgium investigated the possibility of eradication by a combination of antibiotic-based drugs (similar to Hp) and the effect of vaccines using urease or whole cells (158, 162, 163). In South Korea, the infection status of *H. heilmannii* and *H. suis* in pigs and the reproducibility of mouse infection experiments were also examined (159, 167). There are many case reports of MALT lymphoma in South Korea and China, and this is thought to be due to the large number of livestock kept there and eating habits that will be discussed below.

In Japan, the formation of gastric MALT lymphoma caused by Hp and its immunological mechanism have been investigated using thymectomized mice at Kyoto University (described later) (161). In addition, Ota and Katsuyama *et a*l. of Shinshu University examined a large number of cases that were positive for human *H. heilmannii* and *H. suis*, and reported that there were many positive cases for gastric MALT lymphoma (8); the formation of lesions was confirmed by infecting the Mongolian gerbils. More recently, Ota and Katsuyama *et al.* recently revealed the specificity of high endothelial venules in gastric MALT lymphoma (171).

The authors' research findings

In 1998, we collaborated with Shinichi Takahashi (Department of Internal Medicine, Kyorin University) and Takeshi Ito (Tokyo Microscope Institute): gastric mucosal homogenate from crab-eating monkeys was passed on to C3H mice as urease-positive bacteria. It was confirmed that this bacterium was *H. heilmannii*, and it was registered in the DDBJ (DNA data bank of Japan) as *Candidatus* Helicobacter heilmannii TKY. The long-term infection of C57BL / 6 mice with this bacterium forms a small, round and elevated lesion on the mucosa of the gastric glands (which is a characteristic of MALT lymphoma), consisting mainly of an accumulation of B lymphocyte-based lymphocytes and centrocyte-like cells as well as plasma cells.

The presence of severe lymphopepithelial lesions (LEL) was reported as a characteristic of gastric MALT lymphoma (Figs. 20, 21). This bacterium may not be completely eradicated by the primary eradication method using a combination of an antibiotic and a PPI as used for Hp. This MALT lymphoma has strong vascular endothelial growth factor (VEGF) immunoreactivity and relevant receptors, i.e. Flt-1, Flt-3, and Flk-1. It was reported that a mixed administration of the antibodies or inhibitors against these receptors had a significant reduction effect (164-166, 168).

Fig. 20 MALT lymphoma formation in *H. suis* long-term infected C57BL / 6 mice (macroscopic observation)

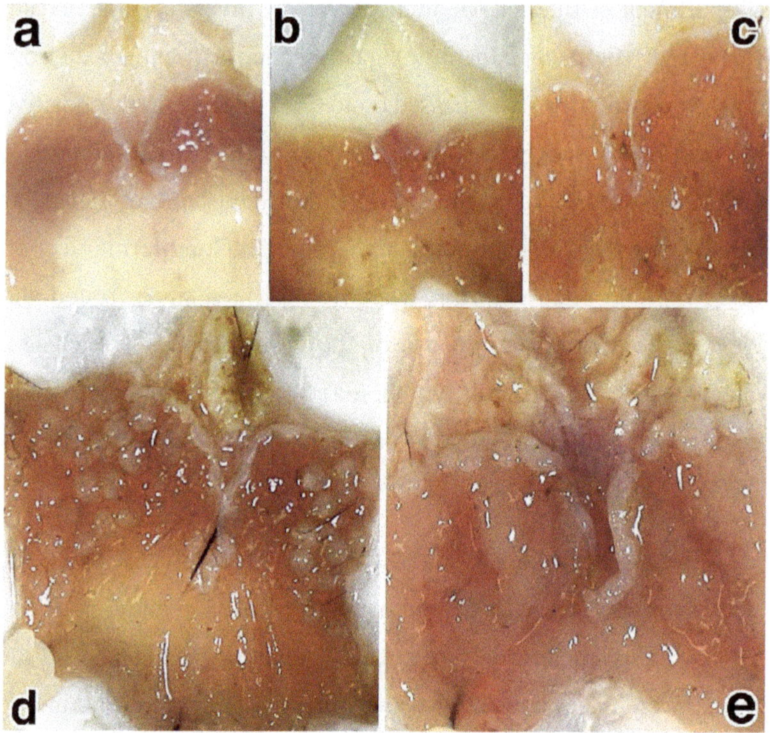

Small, round and elevated lesions are formed in the body of the stomach. They gradually grow in size and merges. a: Control group. b: 3 months later. b: 6 months later. c: 12 months later. d: 18 months later.

Figure 21 Formation of MALT lymphoma in Histology

It is initially recognized as a collection of lymphocytes in the lamina propria just above the muscularis mucosae (a). It gradually progresses to the mucosal layer and submucosal layer (b). Lymphoepithelial lesions and erosions on the tip of the mucosa are also observed (c, d).

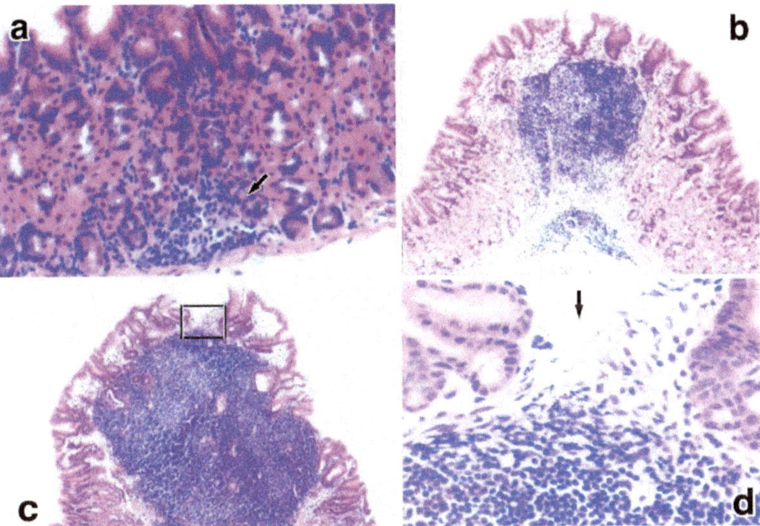

There are some issues with this experimental system. The first question is whether it is so-called follicular gastritis that remains in lymphoid formation or is more advanced, i.e., whether it remains mucosa-associated lymphoid tissue (MALT) or has progressed to MALT lymphoma. In this regard, it is important to examine the presence of BCL-2, BCL-X, and monoclonality by IgH, etc., but the pathological determination of whether or not there is a high degree of LEL is considered to be the most important.

The relationship between gastric NHPH and lymphoma grade

The grading of MALT lymphoma is also important in comparisons with clinical cases. Many reports have shown that longer observation periods reduce the proportion of low grades and increase that of high grades. In this regard, proliferating cell nuclear antigen (PCNA) immunoactivity is thought to be of some help, as in clinical cases. There are few reports on the association of gastric NHPH with advancement into diffuse large B cell lymphoma (DLBCL) in animals, and thus a detailed follow-up is considered necessary in the future.

Relationship between gastric NHPH and chromosomal translocation .

Clinical reports have indicated that chromosomal translocation is related to prognosis, but opposite results also exist. It is difficult to clarify the significance of chromosomal translocation in animal experiments because the chromosomal changes in humans that correspond to those in animals are not known.

Problems when comparing animal lesions with human lesions

Among experimental mouse strains, BALB / c mice are more susceptible to Th2 activation against foreign antigens and infections compared to murine strains such as C3H / HeN and C57BL / 6. This is one of the reasons why BALB / C mice have been frequently used in experimental systems for MALT lymphoma formation. However, as evidenced by our studies and Park's review (160), there are findings suggesting that C57BL / 6 mice are more likely to form lymphoma in gastric MALT lymphoma caused by gastric NHPH. In our gastric NHPH infection experiments using interleukin (IL)-10 knockout mice, lymphoma formation was suppressed, which, as Park *et al.* pointed out, emphasizes the importance of Th2 cytokines.

In this regard, a study of thymectomized BALB / c mice from a group at Kyoto University is interesting (161). In normal Th2-dominant mice, gastric MALT lymphoma was not formed, whereas in the thymectomized group, TH1was predominant, and when infection was added, Th2 became involved and lymphoma was formed. It is necessary to clarify the underlying mechanisms in more detail, not only from the viewpoint of the Th1 and Th2 balance.

MALT lymphoma is thought to be caused by a multi-step process, and its immunological mechanisms are being investigated

(162, 163). It will be informative to study various genetically modified animals, and future progress is expected.

Effect of vagal nerve dissection

In recent years, crosstalk between tumor cells and nerves has been attracting attention in prostate cancer (164), gastric cancer (165), and breast cancer (166). A proposed mechanism is that tumor cells promote nerve cell formation, and the activation of muscarinic receptors promotes cell transformation; i.e., tumorigenesis and tumor progression from stem cells and progenitor cells. Chun-Mei *et al.* investigated the relationship between the onset of gastric cancer and vagal dissection using the INS-GAS mouse model, which is a spontaneous gastric cancer model, and found gastric cancer in 14% on the anterior wall where vagal dissection was performed, and 76% developed gastric cancer on the posterior wall (167). They also reported that tumorigenesis was suppressed in muscarinic m3 receptor knockout mice, and that Wnt was involved in these mechanisms.

For the purpose of examining the involvement of the vagal nerve in the formation of gastric MALT lymphoma, our colleague Yosuke Kodama performed truncal vagal nerve dissection (UVT) of the left branch of the abdominal esophageal vagal nerve of the gastric NHPH-infected mice, and the formation of MALT lymphomas in the isolated gastric anterior wall and posterior wall and the number of bacteria were compared (168). As a result, there was no difference in the number of bacteria or the number of lymphomas, but the lymphomas were significantly larger on the anterior wall where UVT was performed. On the other hand, the thickness of the stomach wall became thinner at the anterior wall, demonstrating the effect of UVT. The formation of follicles, which is considered to be a precursor lesion of lymphoma, was increased in the posterior wall (Fig. 22). The focus of histochemical studies was the localization of substance P-positive nerve fibers. These fibers were increased around the lymphoma on the anterior wall where UVT was performed, and this had a strong effect on mesenchymal cells, suggesting their involvement (Fig. 6). Regarding the relationship between vagal nerve dissection and substance P, it has been reported that substance P increases due to vagal nerve dissection in breast cancer (169), which is consistent with this finding in mice.

Figure 22 History of vagal dissection and the effect of unilateral vagal dissection on gastric MALT lymphoma formation

a: Experimental schedule for unilateral vagal dissection. b: HE staining reveals significantly promoted MALT lymphoma formation at the anterior wall in both pre- and post-infection groups. c: There was no significant difference in the bacterial count by PCR. d: There was no significant difference in the number of MALT lymphomas between the anterior and posterior walls.

Year	Author	Content
1902	Pavlov	analysis of cephalic phase of gastric acid secretion in experiment
1917	Dragstedt	suppression of gastroduodenal ulcer by vagotomy in experiment
1920	Brandt	distribution of vagal nerve
1922	Latarjet	start of vagotomy in clinical medicine
1942	Dragstedt	suppression of gastroduodenal ulcer by vagotomy in clinical medicine, and many modification
		:
2014	Zhao	suppression of experimental gastric ulcer by unilateral vagotomy

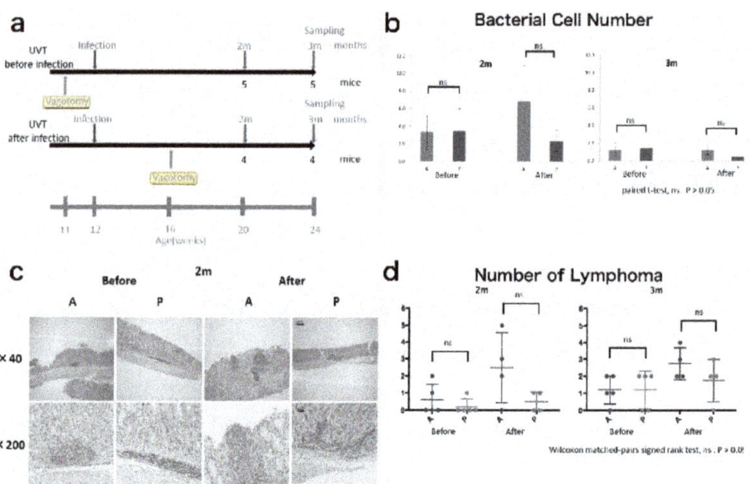

Chapter 10 The association with diseases other than in the digestive tract

Helicobacter pylori **infection is reported to be associated with diseases in organs other than the gastrointestinal tract, and gastric NHPH is also reported to be associated with extragastric diseases. MALT lymphoma of the liver and lung is discussed next.**

During the study of gastric long-term NHPH-infected mice, we observed that MALT lymphoma similar to those located in the stomach were formed in the liver and lung (Fig. 23) (181).

Figure 23 Liver, lung and gastric MALT lymphoma in long-term *H. suis*-infected C57BL / 6 mice. H&E staining.

Top: Liver, Middle: Lung, Bottom: Stomach

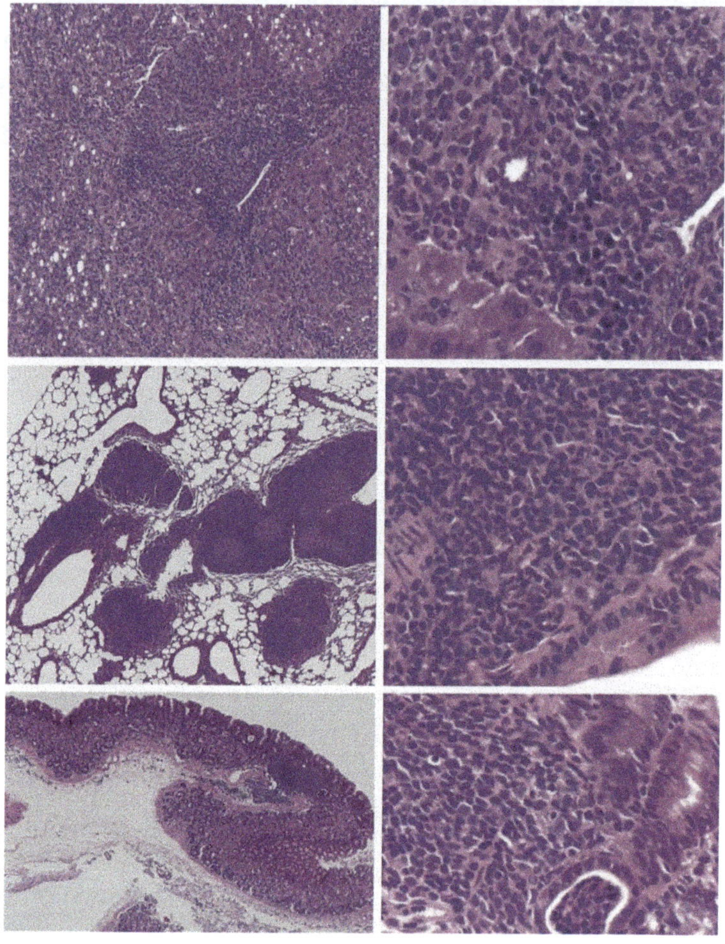

Mechanism and classification of hepatic lymphomas

Liver lymphoma (primary hepatic lymphoma: PHL) is a non-Hodgkin lymphoma (NHL) and is considered extremely rare, but secondary liver lymphoma is quite common; in addition, 40% of NHLs have liver metastases. (182). Viral infections such as hepatitis B virus (HBV) and hepatitis C virus (HCV) and autoimmune diseases such as systemic lupus erythematosus (SLE) are suspected to be involved in PHL, but it is not clear whether they are mere comorbidities or have a causal relationship. The number of reports of PHL associated with HCV has been gradually increasing (183).

The underlying mechanism is thought to be that HCV stimulates B cells, causing monoclonal B cell proliferation and then monoclonal proliferation, and it is speculated that Bcl2 and monoclonal IgH proliferation are involved in the process, and that the same process also occurs in HBV (183).

Pathologically, it has been reported that diffuse large B-cell lymphoma (DLBCL) is the most common hepatic lymphoma, and Burkitt lymphoma and T-cell lymphoma are also found (184), but MALT lymphoma is the second most common lymphoma type. It is said to account for 40% of PHL cases (185).

The relationship between hepatic lymphoma and autonomic nervous system, substance P

The long-term infection of C57BL/6 mice with gastric NHPH causes the formation of MALT lymphoma in the lung and liver that are similar to those observed in the stomach, although the formation takes a longer time than in the stomach (186). The progress over time is shown in Figure 24. The transition route from stomach to liver to lungs is thought be through the vascular system, but the lymphatic system could also be involved because many immature lymphatics were recognized in the surrounding area of the MALT lymphoma (182).

Fig. 24 Time course of gastric, liver, and lung MALT lymphoma formation in long-term *H. suis*-infected C57BL/6 mice

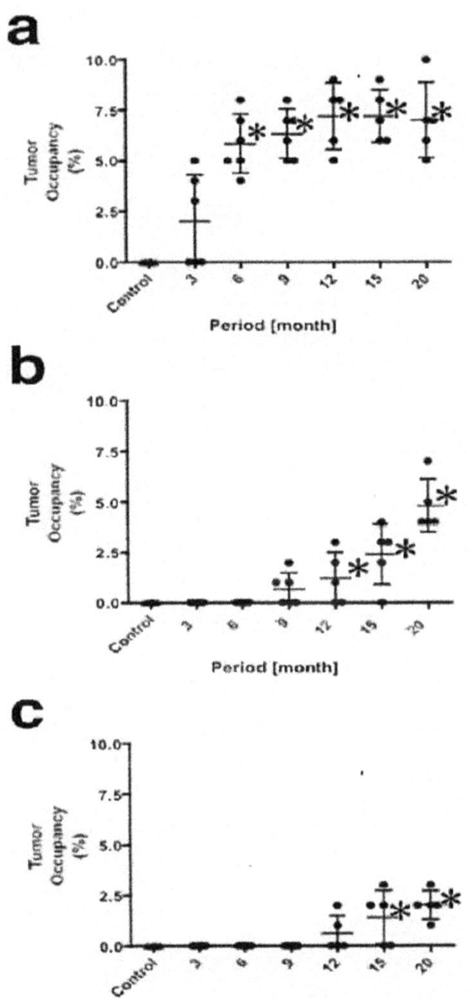

In the histochemical examination, B lymphocytes were accumulated mainly in the stomach, liver, and lung, and gastric NHPHs were scattered within the MALT lymphoma as revealed by the *in situ* hybridization method (Fig. 25).

Fig. 25 Distribution of cells in stomach, liver, and lung in long-term *H. suis*-infected C57BL/6 mice by *in situ* hybridization method

a, b: Stomach. c, d: Liver. e, f: Lung

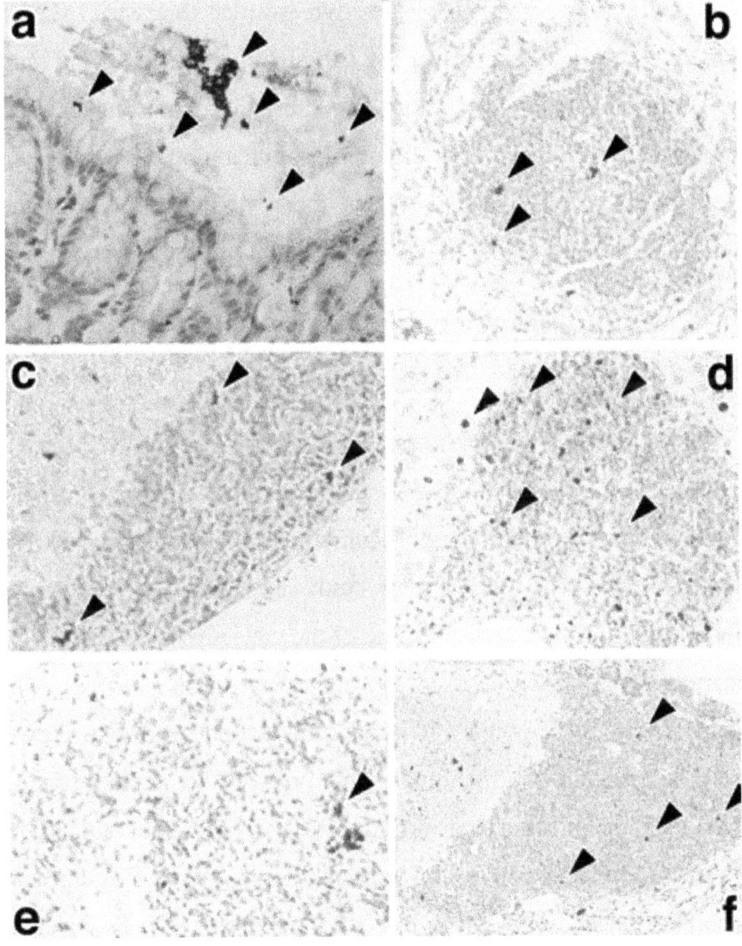

This finding was obtained by Ota *et al.*, and they also investigated the relationship between the MALT lymphoma and the MadCAM-1-positive high endothelial venules as mentioned above (172). The elucidation of this relationship between the two will also help clarify the pathogenesis of the MALT lymphoma. Many of the tumor cells were substance P-positive, similar to gastric MALT lymphoma (186). These findings suggest that gastric, liver, and lung MALT lymphomas have similar characteristics. The translocation of the bacteria themselves is thought to be hematogenous between the stomach and liver and between the liver and lungs, but the possibility of lymphocyte translocation cannot be ruled out.

The association between gastric NHPH and pulmonary lymphoma

Lung MALT lymphoma, also known as pMALToma or bronchial-associated lymphoid tissue lymphoma, is associated with Sjögren's syndrome, infected rheumatism, collagen disease, Hp infection, and AIDS (177). Our study indicated that long-term infection with gastric NHPH is one of the causes of this tumor, and our mouse model can be used as a model of disease formation in humans (171). Substance P and its receptor NK-1R were also shown to be distributed in this tumor, and one of the antagonists of substance P (spantide II) was found to have a tumor-reducing effect (178), which was also observed with another substance P antagonist, aprepitant. These findings are consistent with reports that substance

P has a tumor-suppressing effect (179), and it is drawing attention as a potential new treatment for these tumors.

Gastric, liver, and lung MALT lymphomas in clinical cases

When considering the clinical significance of gastric NHPH, the question of whether or not a similar pathological condition is formed in humans is important.

Iida *et al.* reported a case of liver MALT lymphoma discovered during surgery in a patient with Hp-positive early gastric cancer (180). A patient in whom a liver MALT lymphoma was pathologically diagnosed as cholangiocarcinoma after surgery of liver lesions was described by Dong *et al.* (181), and erosive gastritis was identified by an endoscopic search. However, in that patient, Hp was not detected by the standard test. A patient with a coexisting lung MALT lymphoma and gastric MALT lymphoma was reported by Yanai *et al.* (194), and lung lesions were observed in the patient 8 months after radiotherapy for the gastric MALT lymphoma; an immunohistochemical examination revealed the lung MALT lymphoma. The relationship between gastric and lung lesions is unknown, but this case should be noted.

The relationships among liver tumors, lung tumors, autonomic nerves, and neuropeptides were described briefly above, especially concerning MALT lymphomas. In addition to the importance of the careful observation of clinical cases, experimental systems can provide important information about disease-formation mechanisms and treatment methods.

Chapter 11 Cats and dogs as pets, pigs as livestock and gastric NHPH

Gastric NHPH-related disease is zoonotic, and there have been sporadic reports of transmission from pets and livestock to humans. There are significant differences in pet ownership rates and breeding methods depending on the country, but epidemiological studies suggest a relationship with gastric NHPH. The need for eradication of bacterial infections and drug treatments of pets and livestock remain an important challenge.

The term "companion animal" has come to be used to describe animals who are not only pets but also life companions, and the term also reflects humans' deeper feelings towards animals in captivity, especially with the aging and declining birthrate of some societies in recent years (Fig. 26). Some companion animals are treated like humans

(http://www.inuyanekotachi.com/juku/backnum/201103/).

Keeping dogs and cats as pets, and the link to bacterial infections

Figure 26 What is a companion animal?

In the editorial of the first issue of the *Journal of Animal Ethics* (back in the ancient year 2011), the editors ask prospective authors to replace the word 'pet' with the word 'companion animal:

Specifically, we are inviting authors to use "companion animals" rather than "pets." Despite its prevalence, "pets" is surely a derogatory term with respect to both the animals concerned and their human caregivers.

However, some ethicists quickly pointed out that equating the terms would gloss over the differences.

To quickly illustrate the main point:

You *own* a pet.

You *live with* a companion animal.

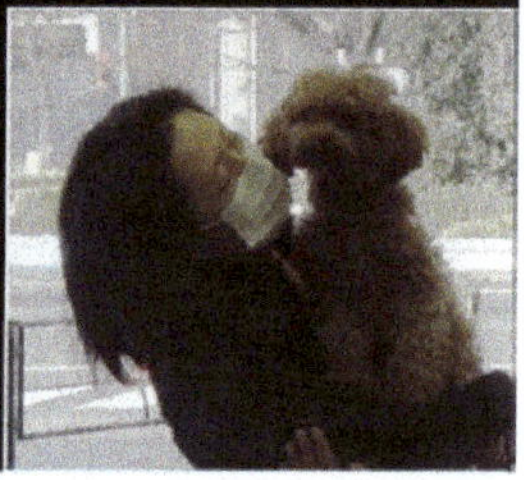

Before examining the relationship between companion animals and livestock and gastric NHPH, the world's pet ownership rate shown in Figure 27 should be noted, with the largest number of pets being kept in Central and South America. Approximately 80% of people in Argentina and Mexico and 75% in Brazil have pets. Russia (73%) and the United States (70%) follow the three Latin American countries. The pet rate is much lower in three Asian countries, with South Korea at 31%, Hong Kong at 35%, and Japan at 37%. On the other hand, in terms of the number of animals (Table 20), Japan is the country with the fourth largest number of dogs and the tenth largest number of cats.

Figure 27 Global pet ownership GfK (Growth from Knowledge) research 2018 (https://www.gfk.com/ja/home)

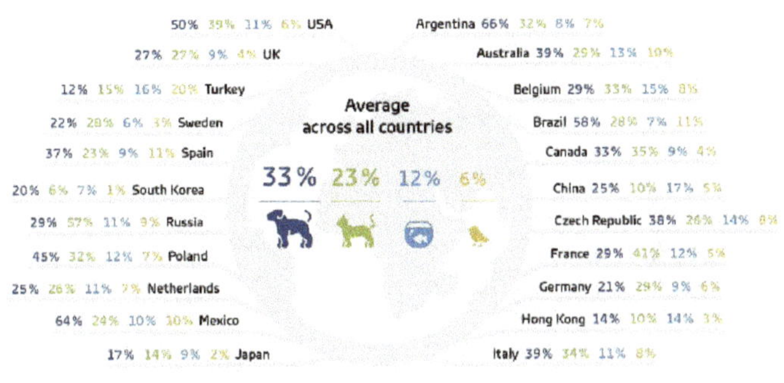

Source: GfK survey among 27,000+ Internet users (ages 15+) in 22 countries – multiple answers possible – rounded

https://www.gfk.com/insights/mans-best-friend-global-pet-ownership-and-feeding-trends

Table 20 The number of dogs and cats in various countries

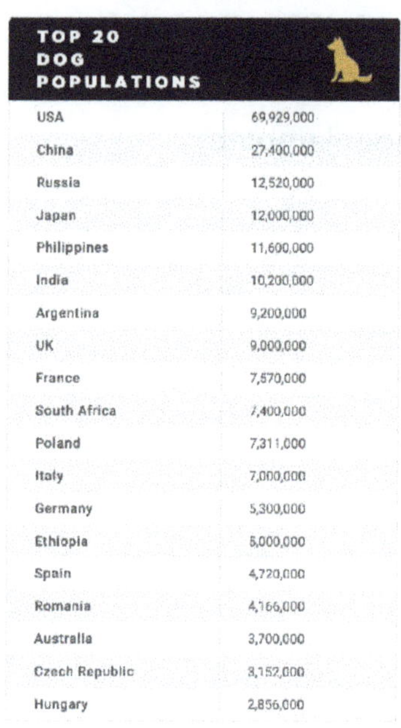

TOP 20 DOG POPULATIONS	
USA	69,929,000
China	27,400,000
Russia	12,520,000
Japan	12,000,000
Philippines	11,600,000
India	10,200,000
Argentina	9,200,000
UK	9,000,000
France	7,570,000
South Africa	7,400,000
Poland	7,311,000
Italy	7,000,000
Germany	5,300,000
Ethiopia	5,000,000
Spain	4,720,000
Romania	4,166,000
Australia	3,700,000
Czech Republic	3,152,000
Hungary	2,856,000

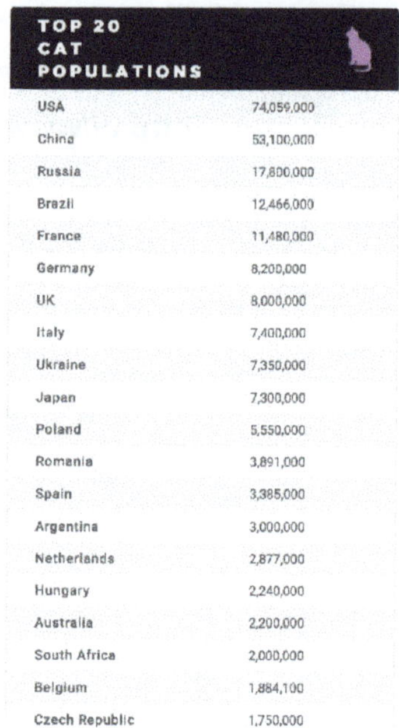

TOP 20 CAT POPULATIONS	
USA	74,059,000
China	53,100,000
Russia	17,800,000
Brazil	12,466,000
France	11,480,000
Germany	8,200,000
UK	8,000,000
Italy	7,400,000
Ukraine	7,350,000
Japan	7,300,000
Poland	5,550,000
Romania	3,891,000
Spain	3,385,000
Argentina	3,000,000
Netherlands	2,877,000
Hungary	2,240,000
Australia	2,200,000
South Africa	2,000,000
Belgium	1,884,100
Czech Republic	1,750,000

Zoonosis and involvement of dogs, cats, pigs, and other animals that are vulnerable to gastric NHPH have been examined.

Regarding zoonotic diseases, it is known that many bacteria belonging to enterohepatic Helicobacter are involved (in addition to gastric NHPH), but only gastric NHPH will be discussed. Table 21 summarizes the reports related to the zoonosis of gastric NHPH. There are many reports from the veterinary field, but only a few will be considered here.

Table 21 Reports related to the zoonosis of gastric NHPH

Year	First Author	Nation	Disease: Gastritis	Nodular Gastritis	Gastric Ulcer	Duodenal Ulcer	MALT Lymphoma	Gastric Cancer	Esophagitis	Others	Species	Relation to zoonosis	Ref Number
1962	Weber AF	Brazil									Spiral organism	EM detection in pig and cat stomach	26
1987	Curry A	UK									Spiral organism	Spiral bacterium in baboon stomach	27
1989	Dye KR	USA	○ 2 cases								Spiro organism	first case keeping 14 cats, second case keeping 2 dogs	28
1990	Mendes EN	Brazil									*Gastrospirillum hominis*	Gastrospirillum hominis in pig stomach	29
1990	Norris CR	USA	○ mild gastritis								*"H. heilmannii"*	high prevalence of "H.heilmannii" in cats, similar to H. felis	
1993	Solnick JV	USA									*H. heilmannii*	named *Gastrospirillum hominis* as *Helicobacter heilmannii*	31
1994	Stolte M	Germany									*H. heilmannii*	Pet keeping rate 70.3% in Hh positive cases, 37% in general population, possibility of Hh as a zoonotic agent [illegible]	195
1994	Lavelle JP	USA	○ 1 case								*G. hominis*	36 yo male using cats for experiment	34
1995	Yang H	China					○ undifferentiated cancer					having history of dog and cat keeping	39
1996	Eaton KA	USA	○ mild to moderate gastritis								*G. hominis or H. felis*	[illegible] 100% in dogs for experiment, 97% in cats	187
1997	Serna JH	USA	E16:E16:N21								HLO	lymph follicle formation in cat mucosa and submucosa, 86% positivity in RUT and UBT	188
1998	Meining A	Germany										pig, cat and dog possible Hh reservoir	186
1998	Neiger R	Switzerland	○									cats Hh 78% positive, but negative to Hp and H felis	189
1999	DeGroote A	Belgium										named *Gastrospirillum suis* as candidatus H. suis	190
2000	Morgner A	Germany					○ 5 cases				*H. heilmannii*	eradication of 5 cases of MALT lymphoma stronger relation than Hp	74
2003	van Loon S	Netherlands	○ 1case								*H. heilmannii*	5 yo boy, keeping two cats, identical gene with cat Hh	79
2004	Priestnall SL	USA										Few Hh type 1 in dogs and cats, many Hh type 1 in human	191
2005	Van den Bulck	Belgium										H. bizzozeronii in dogs, many H. felis, H135 in cats (more than 80%) many human cases	192
2007	Ramis G	Spain										Gradual increase of Hs infection rate in younger generation, influences by antibiotics restriction	193
2007	Nala K	Czechoslovakia	○1case								*H. heilmannii*	17yo male, reinfection 3 years after Hh eradication, improved by gastritis to Hh eradication in pet	58
2010	Jothimani DK	UK	○ 1case								*H. heilmannii*	37yo female, keeping cat	[illegible]
2013	Foss DL	USA										half of pigs positive to Hs	194
2017	Tsukadaira T	Japan	○ 9 cases								NHPH	dog keeping in 5 cases, cat keeping in one case, no relation to pigs	103
2018	Nakagawa S	Japan	○ 1case								*H. suis*	56 yo male, not dog pig keeping history	104
2020	Nakamura M	Japan	○ 36 cases	○ 6 cases	○ 2 cases	○ 1 case	○ 11case			Sjogren synd 1case	NHPH	higher NHPH in higher pork consumption area	107
2020	Shafaie S	Iran	○ 17cases		25 cases	○ 17cases					NHPGH	few cases with H bizzozeroni, possibly related to low pet keeping rate in Iran	108

zoonosis
dog, cat
pig
others

Stolte *et al.* examined contact with livestock that triggered the transmission of gastric NHPH to humans, and 111 (70.3%) of the 125 positive humans had contact with animals (195). Since the contact rate with animals in general population is 37%, the possibility of infection from livestock and pets is thought to be high. In addition, since the mixed infection rate of Hp and gastric NHPH is very low, the possibility that gastric NHPH infection may prevent Hp infection was pointed out. A subsequent epidemiological study from the same group (196) reported that pigs, cats, and dogs were reservoirs of gastric NHPH infection. Researchers also described as developing gastritis and gastric ulcers due to the gastric NHPH transmitted from cats.

Recent studies have reported that *H. heilmannii* was found in dogs, cats, primates, pigs, rodents, and rabbits. However, when considering the relationship between humans and animals, many infected people have had pets in the past but not currently, and the problem is that we cannot distinguish between past and recent infections. Table 23 lists natural hosts other than humans and their characteristics, and Figure 28 describes points to note when living with pets.

Table 22 Characteristics of gastric Helicobacter bacteria reported for zoonosis

Helicobacter	Species	Natural host	Length (mm)	Width (mm)	Flagella	Periplasmic fibrils	GC content (mol%)
gastric NHPH	*H. bizzozeronii*	Cat, dog, fox, lynx	5-10	0.3	bipolar	No	46
	H. felis	Cat, dog, rabbit, cheetah	5-7.5	0.4	bipolar	Yes	42
	H. heilmannii ss	Cat, dog, fox, lynx, non-human primates	3-6.5	0.6-0.7	bipolar	No	47.4
	H. salomonis	Cat, dog, rabbit	5-7	0.8-1.2	bipolar	No	
	H. suis	Pig, non-human primates	2.3-6.7	0.9-1.2	bipolar	No	39.9
H.pylori		Human, non-human primates	2.5-5	0.5-1	unipolar	No	39

Figure 28 Points to note about living with pets

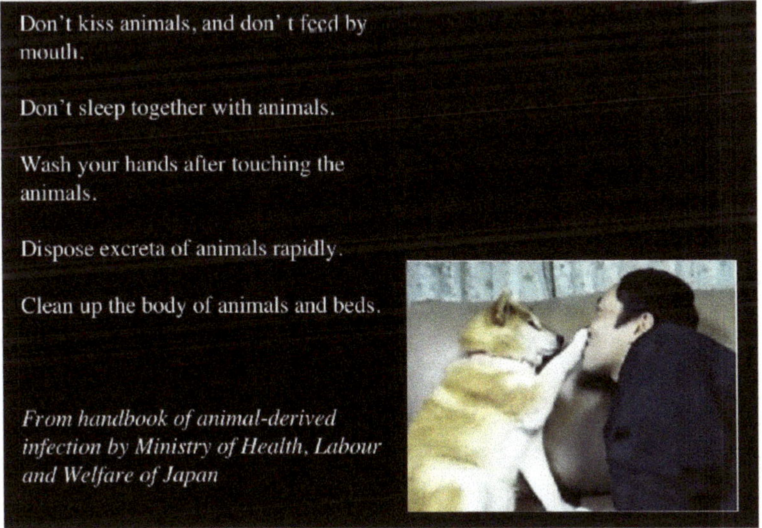

The relationship between gastric NHPH and pigs

There are many recent reports that *H. suis* accounts for more than half of human cases of gastric NHPH infections, and it has been noted that pigs as meat rather than pets may be involved, mentioned above in Chapter 6. We reported results that agree with the idea from the distribution in Japan.

In Fig 29, the number of breeding animals in China is shown to be overwhelmingly large, and it is likely that there are many cases of *H. suis* infection in China.

Fig 29 Number of pigs raised worldwide

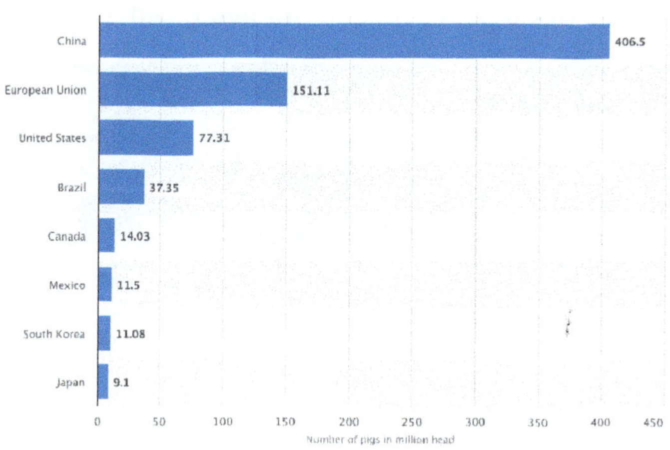

https://www.statista.com/statistics/263964/number-of-pigs-in-selected-countries/

Looking at the infection rate of pigs, a U.S. study reported that more than half of the pigs examined were affected (204). In terms of eating habits, it has been reported that the infection rate is high in areas such as northeastern China (97) and Belgium (205) where raw pork stomach or meat is eaten as it is or in paste form.

Even in Japan, although the pork meat is not raw, there is a habit of eating the stomach of pork as one of the grilled offal, so it seems that its involvement cannot be denied (Fig. 30).

Figure 30 Name of pig part in grilled offal

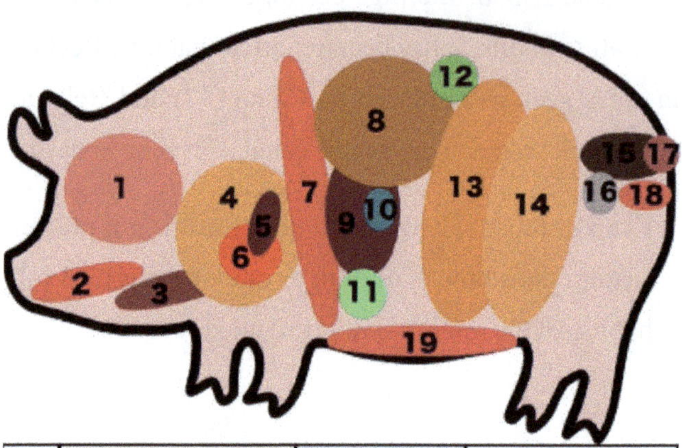

	Japanese Offal Name	Organ name	Good for Beginner
1	Kashira	cheek	○
2	Butatan (Tontan)	tongue	○
3	Nankotsu	throat	○
4	Fuwa	lung	
5	Hatsumoto	aorta	
6	Hatsu	heart	○
7	Butaharami	diaphragm	○
8	Gatsu	stomach	
9	Lebar	liver	
10	Shibire	pancreas	
11	Chire	spleen	
12	Mame	kidney	
13	Shiro	small intettine	
14	Shirokoro	large intestine	
15	Teppou	rectum	
16	Kobukuro	uterus	
17	Dote	anus	
18	Rappa	vagina	
19	Oppai	breast	

The relationship between the gastric NHPH and the history of domestication

The history of domestication or domestication of animals by humans is said to have started with dogs roughly 15,000 to 36,000 years ago, depending on the age when a dog was observed to have been buried with a person or depicted in painting. Farming is estimated to have begun 10,000 years ago, and from that time, the domestication of herbivores such as sheep, goats, cattle and pigs began (206).

Figure 31 The history of the domestication of animals (206)

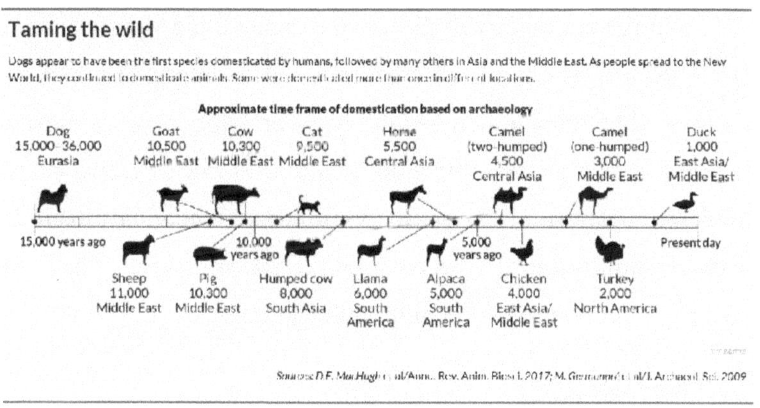

As described in Chapter 6, in 2017 Flahou *et al.* reported gastric NHPH-infected pigs from non-human primates between 100,000 and 15,000 years ago, after which the domestication of pigs occurred. They suggested that the infection occurred sporadically and revealed that it had a completely different evolutionary pathway from Hp (148). In addition, since *H. suis* is not found in wild boar, it is suspected that *H. suis* infection occurred between the differentiation of wild boar into pigs and the domestication of pigs.

Regarding the wolf, which is considered to be the ancestor of dogs, gastric NHPH has not been identified in wolves (Table 22). This is an interesting issue because it is related to the time of the differentiation from wolves to dogs.

The relation to emerging and re-emerging infectious disease and one health approach

In the era of Covid-19, we must realize the significance of gastric NHPH as one of the emerging and re-emerging infectious diseases, although not included in Fig 32 probably because most of these diseases are acute infection, while influence of Helicobacter infection is chronic. 70% of emerging and re-emerging infectious diseases show vector-borne or zoonotic transmission. Thus, we must pay attention to the relation to the animals.

Fig. 32

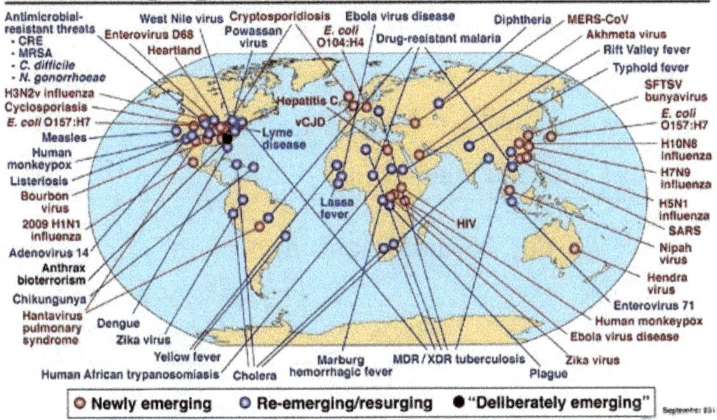

https://www.niaid.nih.gov/sites/default/files/main%20map.jpg

The concept of one health must also be considered from the similar connotation. One Health is an approach that recognizes that the health of people is closely connected to the health of animals and our shared environment. One Health has become more important in recent years. This is because many factors have changed interactions between people, animals, plants, and our environment. We must also estimate the significance of NHPH infection, especially how to be in contact with companion animals and livestock from this point of view (Fig.33).

Fig. 33 one health approach

One Health
Coordinating
Communicating
Collaborating
People who protect human, animal, and environmental health, and other partners
To achieve the best health outcomes for people, animals, plants, and our environment
CDC
Centers for Disease Control and Prevention
National Center for Emerging and Zoonotic Infectious Diseases

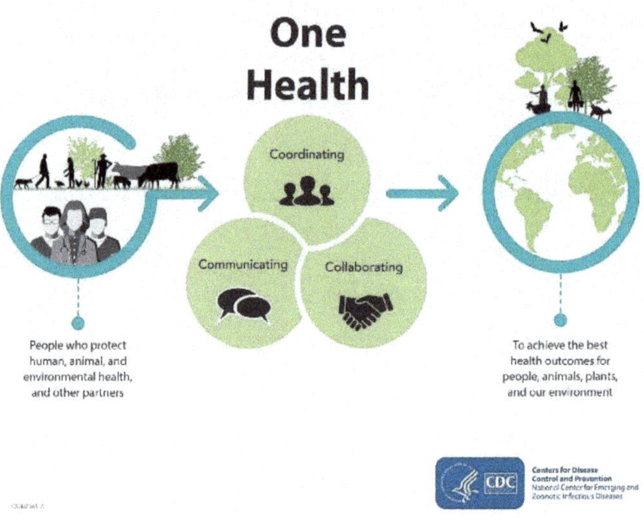

https://www.cdc.gov/onehealth/images/multimedia/one-health-def.jpg

Chapter 12 Future tasks

Simply inciting fear of zoonosis is unscientific; evidence-based results will lead to the further development of our knowledge of Helicobacter in humans and animals.

The significance of Hp in the formation of upper gastrointestinal disease and the current information about the association between these diseases and gastric NHPH can be summarized as follows.

The main theory of the significance of Hp in upper gastrointestinal diseases has been regarded as something like a "central dogma" stating that "many upper gastrointestinal diseases are exclusively caused by *Helicobacter pylori*". The following are point to consider, especially concerning future tasks in this field of research.

1. There are some cases of Hp-negative nodular gastritis, which is considered an initial infection with Hp.

This point can already be explained by gastric NHPH, as described herein, but since gastric NHPH has been observed in 30% of the

Hp-negative nodular gastritis cases., one can surmise that gastric NHPH is involved.

2. The ABC classification is based on anti-Hp antibody titer and pepsinogen I/II ratio for the estimation of the healthy balance of the stomach. The reliability of the ABC classification is high, but there are 10%-20% cases with gastritis in the normal group A, and they are classified into group pseudo-A.

These cases include patients who used to be infected with Hp and underwent Hp eradication with the intake of antibiotics for some other infection, but it is thought that these cases also include gastric NHPH infection, in which the serum Hp antibody is negative.

3. The MALT lymphoma cases showing Hp-positivity are treated with eradication therapy, but even in Hp-negative MALT lymphoma cases Hp eradication sometimes induces the resolution of the tumors.　This may be explained by the immunomodulatory effect of antibacterial agents, but as described above, it is more likely to think that some of these Hp-negative gastric MALT lymphoma cases may be caused by gastric NHPH.

4. Will microbial substitution take place in the stomach after Hp eradication? In Japan, the Hp of more than 1 million people is eradicated annually.

As in the case of nontuberculous mycobacteriosis of the lung after the eradication of tuberculosis, we must keep in mind that infection with gastric NHPH or other bacteria could increase after eradication of *Helicobacter pylori*. This has not yet been documented, but it may have occurred already.

Chapter 13 Conclusion Gastric NHPH and Helicobacter pylori Similarities with the 10th planet

When thinking about gastric NHPH, I sometimes remember the science fiction story "The 10th Planet" that I read as a kid.

In this story, there is another planet on the other side of the sun, and its existence had not been known, but on that planet similar human beings live there as well.

Although the existence of this tenth planet is now scientifically denied, in the story the Earth and this planet are secretly but always influencing each other.

Applying this story to *Helicobacter pylori* and gastric NHPH, one can think of gastric NHPH as a 'tenth planet', and only a part of its characteristics have been clarified. As to the size of its influence, is it negligibly small or unexpectedly large for *Helicobacter pylori* corresponding to the Earth? Is the relationship between Hp and gastric NHPH a predator-prey relationship, a competitive relationship, a symbiotic relationship, or a parasitic relationship ?

By the time gastric NHPH was discovered, it was proposed

that this bacterium in pets could suppress the settlement of *Helicobacter pylori* on the human gastric mucosa and is beneficial to humans, and that NHPH is a bacterium that enhances the significance of pets' existence. However, the relationship between gastric cancer and gastric NHPH (which is considered to be the most important) is not well understood, and the true clinical weighting of this bacterium is still unknown.

The reports that have accumulated worldwide are summarized herein, ant it is hoped that we will be able to meet new challenges in future academic conferences and treatises.

We thank Tetsufumi Takahashi, Yukie Sekiya, Yosuke Kodama for their hard work and Dr. Hiroshi Michimae for the help with statistical processing. We would also like to express our deep gratitude to all the graduates of the School of Pharmacy, Kitasato University (who became the driving force of the present research with their youthful enthusiasm), the many other people concerned, and the family members whose patience is much appreciated.

In April 2021, in the Covid-19 era, ··

Authors ····································

Memory of NHPH, bacterial "tenth planet"

I still remember very well,
the day I finally found the bacteria I had wanted to see avidly for many years.
The bacteria had been concealed in the secret niche of the mucus layer,
but I could see the spiral bacteria by the electron microscopy suddenly.
The bacteria was gradually lost in the dark by the destruction of the embedding resin by the strong electron beam.

Good bye, my NHPH!
But I am still very happy
because I actually watched you with my own eyes.

References

Chapter 1 Looking back on our research group's 20-years history

1) Itoh T, Yanagawa Y, Singaki M, Masubuchi N, Takahashi S & Saito S. Isolation of *Helicobacter Heilmannii* like organism from the stomachs of cynomolgus monkeys and colonization of them in mice. Gastroenterology, 106 (Suppl), A99, 1994.

Chapter 2 NHPH Nomenclature

2) Muller OF. Animacula infusoria fluviatilia et marina, quae detexit, systematice descript et ad vivum delineari. Huaniae, N. Molleri, 1786.

3) Ehrenberg CG. Die Infusionsthierchen als vollkommene Organismen. Leipzig, Voss, 1838.

4) Bottcher G: Dorpater Med Z 1875;184.

5) Rappin J. Contre a l'etude de bacteri de la bouche a l' et at normal.1881; 68. Quoted by Breed RS, Murray EGD, Hitchens AP. Bergey's manual of determinative bacteriology, 6th ed. Baltimore: Williams and Wilkins Co, 1948: 217.

6) Jaworski W. Podrecznik Chorob zoladka. Wy- dawnictwa Dziel Lekarskich Polskich 1889;32.

7) Bizzozero G. Ueber die schlauchformigen drusen desmagendarmkanals und die beziehungen ihres epithels zu demoberflachenepithel der schleimhaut. Archivfur MikrofkopischeAnatomie Entwickiungs mechanik 42: 82, 1893.

8) Salomon H. Ueber das spirillum des saugetiermagens und seinverhalten zu den belegzellen. Centralblatt fur Bakteriologie,Parasitenkunde V. Infektionskrankheiten XIX: 433-43, 1896.

9) Kasai K, Kobayashi R. The stomach spirochete occurring in mammals. J. Parasitol. 6: 1-11, 1919.

10) Doenges JL. Spirochaetes in gastric glands of Macacus rhesus and humans without definite history of related disease. Proc Soc Exp Biol Med 1938;38:536–538, 1938.

11) Palmer ED. Investigation of the gastric mucosa spirochetes of the human. Gastroenterology 1954;27:218–220, 1954.

12) Edkins JS. Spirella regaudi in the cat. Parasitology 1923;15:296–307, 1923.

13) Modlin IM, Sachs G, Wright N, Kidd M. Edkins and a century of acid suppression. Digestion. 2005;72(2-3):129-45, 2005.

14) Luck JM. Gastric urease. Biochem J 18: 1227–1231, 1924.

15) Conway EJ. The Biochemistry of Gastric Acid Secretion. Springfield, Thomas, 1952.

16) Kornberg HL; Davies RE. Gastric urease. Physiol Rev 35:169–177, 1955.

17) Steer HW. Ultrastructure of cell migration through the gastric epithelium and its relation- ship to bacteria. J Clin Pathol 28:639–646, 1975.

18) Ramsey EJ, Carey KV, Peterson WL, Jackson JJ, Murphy FK, Read NW, Taylor KB, Trier JS, Fordtran JS. Epidemic gastritis with hypochlorhydria. Gastroenterology 76: 1449–1457, 1979.

19) Graham DY, Alpert LC, Smith JL, Yoshimura HH. Iatrogenic *Campylobacter pylori* infection is a cause of epidemic achlorhydria. Am J Gastroenterol 83:974–980, 1988.

20) Marshall BJ; Warren JR. Unidentified curved bacilli in the stomach of patients with gastritis and peptic ulceration. Lancet vol. 1(8390) p. 1311-5, 1984.

21) Marshall BJ, Armstrong JA, McGechie DB, Glancy RJ. Attempt to fulfill Koch's postulates for pyloric campylobacter. Med J Aust 142:436–439, 1985.

Chapter 3 History of gastric NHPH research

22) Dent JC, McNulty CA, Uff JC, Wilkinson SP, Gear MW. Spiral organisms in the gastric antrum. Lancet Jul 11; 2(8550): 96-96, 1987.

23） McNulty CA, Dent JC, Curry A, Uff JS, Ford GA, Gear MW & Wilkinson SP. New spiral bacterium in gastric mucosa. J Clin Pathol, 42, 585-591, 1989.

24）Heilmann KL, Nowottny U. Histologischer Nachweis von CLO (Campylobacter Like Organisms) in Magenbiopsien. Dtsch Med Wochenschr; 112: 861-862, 1987.

25） Heilmann KL, Borchard F. Gastritis due to spiral shaped bacteria other than *Helicobacter pylori*: clinical, histological, and ultrastructural findings. Gut, 32:137-40, 1991.

26） Weber AF, Schmittdiel EF. Electron microscopic and bacteriologic studies of spirilla isolated from the fundic stomachs of cats and dogs. Am J Vet Res 23:422-7, 1962.

27） Curry A, Jones DM, Eldridge J. Spiral organisms in the baboon stomach. Lancet ii:634-5, 1987.

28） Dye KR, Marshall BJ, Fnerson HF, Onerrant RT, McCall RW. Gastritis in a human due to infection with an organism resembling the cat gastric spirillum. Gastroenterology 1988; 94: A108, 1988.

29) Mendes EN, Queiroz DM, Rocha GA, Moura SB, Leite VH, Fonseca ME. Ultrastructure of a spiral micro-organism from pig gastric mucosa (“*Gastrospirillum suis*”). J. Med. Microbiol. 33: 61-66, 1990.

30) De Groote D, Ducatelle R, Van Doorn LJ, Tilmant K, Quint WGV, Verschuurn A, Haesebrouck F. Detection of “*Candidatus* Helicobacter suis” in gastric samples of pig by PCR: Comparison with other invasive diagnostic techniques. J Clin Microbiol 38: 1131-1135, 2000.

31) Solnick JV, O’Rourke J, Lee A, Paster BJ, Dewhirst FE & Tompkins LS. An uncultured gastric spiral organism is a newly identified Helicobacter in humans. The Journal of infectious diseases, 168: 379-85, 1993.

32) O'Rourke JL, Solnick JV, Lee A, Tompkins LS. *Helicobacter heilmannii* (previously *Gastrospirillum hominis*), a new species of Helicobacter in humans and animals. Ir J Med Sci 161: 31, 1992.

33) De Groote D, van Doorn LJ, Ducatelle R, Verschuuren A, Haesebrouck F, Quint WG, Jalava K, Vandamme P. '*Candidatus* Helicobacter suis', a gastric helicobacter from pigs, and its phylogenetic relatedness to other gastrospirilla. Int J Syst Bacteriol 49 Pt 4: 1769-1777, 1999.

34) O'Rourke JL, Solnick JV, Neilan BA, Seidel K, Hayter R, Hansen LM, Lee A. Description of '*Candidatus* Helicobacter heilmannii' based on DNA sequence analysis of 16S rRNA and urease genes. Int J Syst Evol Microbiol 54: 2203-2211, 2004.

35) Smet A, Flahou B, D'Herde K, Vandamme P, Cleenwerck I, Ducatelle R, Pasmans F, Haesebrouck F. *Helicobacter heilmannii* sp. nov., isolated from feline gastric mucosa. Int J Syst Evol Microbiol 62: 299-306, 2012.

36) Trebesius K, Adler K, Vieth M, Stolte M, Haas R. Specific detection and prevalence of *Helicobacter heilmannii*-like organisms in the human gastric mucosa by fluorescent in situ hybridization and partial DNA sequencing. J .Clin. Microbiol., 39, 1510–1516, 2001.

37) Haesebrouck F, Pasmans F, Flahou B, Smet A, Vandamme P. & Ducatelle R. Non-*Helicobacter pylori* Helicobacter species in the human gastric mucosa: a proposal to introduce the terms *H. heilmannii sensu lato* and *sensu stricto*. Helicobacter, 16: 339–340, 2011.

38) Flahou B, Haesebrouck F, Smet A, Yonezawa H, Osaki T, Kamiya S. Gastric and enterohepatic non-*Helicobacter pylori* Helicobacters. Helicobacter,18 Suppl 1:66-72, 2013.

Chapter 4 Positive cases and positivity rates

39) McNulty CA, Watson DM. Spiral bacteria of the gastric antrum. Lancet 8385:1068-1069, 1984.

40) Heilmann KL. Spirochäten-ähnliche Bakterien in der menschlichen Magenschleimhaut. Dtsch Med Wochenschr. 113:1298－1299, 1988.

41) Dye KR, Marshall BJ, Frierson HF Jr, Guerrant RL, McCallum RW. Ultrastructure of another spiral organism associated with human gastritis. Dig Dis Sci 34:1787–1791, 1989.

42) Figura N, Guglielmetti P, Quaranta S. Spiral shaped bacteria in gastric mucosa. J Clin Pathol 43:173, 1990.

43) Fischer R, Samisch W, Schwenke E. '*Gastrospirillum hominis*': Another four cases. Lancet 335:59, 1990.

44) Morris, A., Ali, M. R., Thomsen, L., & Hollis, B. Tightly spiral shaped bacteria in the human stomach: Another cause of active chronic gastritis? Gut, 31: 139–143, 1990.

45) Flejou JF, Diomande I, Molas G, Goldfain D, Rotenberg A, Florent M, Potet F. Human chronic gastritis associated with non-Helicobacter pylori spiral organisms (*Gastrospirillum hominis*). Four cases and review of the literature. Gastroenterol Clin Biol 14: 808-810, 1990.

46) Borody TJ, George LL, Brandl S, Andrews P, Ostapowicz N, Hyland L, Devine M. *Helicobacter pylori*-negative duodenal ulcer. Am J Gastroenterol 86: 1154-1157, 1991.

47) Nakshabendi IM, Peebles SE, Lee FDRussell RI. Spiral shaped microorganisms in the human duodenal mucosa. Pastgrad Med J 67: 846-847, 1991.

48) Queiroz DMM, Cabral, MMDA, Nogueira AJA, Barbosa AJA, Rocha GA, Mendes EN. Mixed gastric infection by *Gastrospirillum hominis* and *Helicobacter pylori*. Lancet 336: 507-508, 1990.

49) Ierardi E, Monno R, Mongelli A, Allegretta L, Milone E, Rizzi S, Panza P, Coppolecchia P, Francavilla A. *Gastrospirillum hominis* associated chronic active gastritis: the first report from Italy. Ital J Gastroenterol 23: 86-87, 1991.

50) Wegmann W, Aschwanden M, Schaub N, Aenishanslin W, Gyr K. Gastritis associated with *Gastrospirillum hominis* – a zoonosis? Schweiz Med Wochenschr 121:245–254, 1991.

51) Lopez JA, Tamaya MC, Mejia GI, Trujilo H, Espinal D, Perez MA, Robledo JA: *Gastrospirillum hominis* in a child with chronic gastritis. Ped Infect Dis J 12: 701, 1993.

52) Nogueira AM, Ribeiro GM, Rodrigues MA, Queiroz DM, Mendes EN, Rocha GA, Barbosa AJ. Prevalence of *Helicobacter pylori* in Brazilian patients with gastric carcinoma. Am J Clin Pathol 100:236-9, 1993.

53) Mazzucchelli L, Wilder-Smith CH, Ruchti C, Meyer-Wyss B, & Merki HS. *Gastrospirillum hominis* in asymptomatic, healthy individuals. Dig Dis Sci 38: 2087–2089, 1993.

54) Lavelle JP, Landas S, Mitros FA, & Conklin JL. Acute gastritis associated with spiral organisms from cats. Dig Dis Sci 39: 744–750, 1994.

55) Tanaka M, Saitoh A, Narita T, Kudo H. *Gastrospirillum hominis*-associated gastritis: The first reported case in Japan. J Gastroenterol 29: 199-202, 1994.

56) Morgner A, Bayerdorffer E, Meining A, Stolte M, Kroher G. *Helicobacter heilmannii* and gastric cancer. Lancet 346: 511-512, 1995.

57) Hilzenrat N, Lamoureux E, Weintrub I, Alpert E, Lichter M, Alpert L. *Helicobacter heilmannii*-like spiral bacteria in gastric mucosal biopsies. Arch Pathol Lab Med 119:1149-1153, 1995.

58) Akin OY, Tsou VM, & Werner AL. *Gastrospirillum hominis*-associated chronic active gastritis. Pediatr Pathol Lab Med, 15: 429–435, 1995.

59) Yang H, Li X, Xu Z, Zhou D. "*Helicobacter heilmannii*" infection in a patient with gastric cancer. Dig Dis Sci 40: 1013-1014, 1995.

60) Koyanagi M, Tanaka M, Nishi T, *et al.* A case of Gastrospirillum hominis infection with AGML. Itocho, 30:1079-83, 1995. (in Japanese)

61) Debongnie JC, Donnay M, Mairesse J. *Gastrospirillum hominis* ("*Helicobacter heilmannii*"): a cause of gastritis, sometimes transient, better diagnosed by touch cytology? Am J Gastroenterol 90: 411-416, 1995.

62) Stolte M, Kroher G, Meining A, Morgner A, Bayerdörffer E, Bethke B. A comparison of *Helicobacter pylori* and *H. heilmannii* gastritis. A matched control study involving 404 patients. Scand J Gastroenterol. 32: 28-33, 1997.

63) Goddard AF, Logan RP, Atherton JC, Jenkins D, Spiller RC. Healing of duodenal ulcer after eradication of *Helicobacter heilmannii*. Lancet 21;349(9068):1815-6, 1997.

64) Isomoto H, Matsunaga K, *et al*. A case of corpus gastritis with Gastrospirillum hominis infection. Japanese Gastroenterological Endoscopy, 39: 68-72, 1997. (in Japanese)

65)Goteri G, Ranaldi R, Rezai B, Baccarini MG, Bearzi I. Synchronous mucosa-associated lymphoid tissue lymphoma and adenocarcinoma of the stomach. Am J Surg Pathol. 21: 505–509, 1997.

66) Chen Y, Zhou D, Wang J. Biological diagnostic and therapeutic study on the *Helicobacter heilmannii*. Zhonghua Yi Xue Za Zhi. 78: 490-3, 1998.

67) Yali Z, Yamada N, Wen M, Matsuhisa T, Miki M. *Gastrospirillum hominis* and *Helicobacter pylori* infection in Thai individuals: Comparison of histopathological changes of gastric mucosa. Pathol Int 48: 507-511, 1998.

68) Foschini MP, Pieri F, Cerasoli S, Accardo P, Formica G, Biasiucci A, Donzelli C, Villanacci V. *Helicobacter heilmannii*: studio anatomo-clinico di 14 nuovi casi . Pathologica. 91:18-24, 1999.

69) Schultz-Süchting F, Stallmach T, Braegger CP. Treatment of *Helicobacter heilmannii*-associated gastritis in a 14-year-old boy. J Pediatr Gastroenterol Nutr. 28: 341-2, 1999.

70) Jhala D, Jhala N, Lechago J & Haber M. *Helicobacter heilmannii* gastritis: Association with acid peptic diseases and comparison with *Helicobacter pylori* gastritis. Mod Pathol 12: 534–538, 1999.

71) Tiszlavicz L, Suták J, Wittmann T, Cserni G. *Helicobacter heilmannii* (*Gastrospirillum hominis*) asszociált gastritis: az elsö Magyarországon leírt esetek [Helocobacter heilmannii (Gastrospirillum hominis)-associated gastritis: first reported cases in Hungary]. Orv Hetil. 140: 887-90, 1999.

72) Mention K, Michaud L, Guimber D, Martin De Lasalle E, Vincent P, Turck D, Gottrand F. Characteristics and prevalence of *Helicobacter heilmannii* infection in children undergoing upper gastrointestinal endoscopy. J Pediatr Gastroenterol Nutr 29:533-9, 1999.

73) Yamamoto T, Matsumoto J, Shiota K, Kitajima S, Goto M, Imaizumi M, Arima T. *Helicobacter heilmannii* associated erosive gastritis. Intern Med 38: 240-243, 1999.

74) Morgner A, Lehn N, Andersen LP, Thiede C, Bennedsen M, Trebesius K, Neubauer B, Neubauer A, Stolte M, Bayerdorffer E. *Helicobacter heilmannii*-associated primary gastric low-grade MALT lymphoma: complete remission after curing the infection. Gastroenterology 118: 821-828, 2000.

75) Svec A, Kordas P, Pavlis Z, Novotný J. High prevalence of *Helicobacter heilmannii*-associated gastritis in a small, predominantly rural area: further evidence in support of a zoonosis? Scand J Gastroenterol. 35: 925-8, 2000.

76) Kamoshida T, Hotta T, Hirai S, OkaY. A case of antral gastritis with Helicobacter heilmannii infection diagnosed by McMullen method. Japanese Gastroenterological Endoscopy, 42: 974-979, 2000.

77) Ierardi E, Monnro RA, Gentile A, Francavilla R, Burattini O, Marangi S, Pollice L, Francavilla A. *Helicobacter heilmannii* gastritis: A histological and immunohistochemical trait. J Clin Pathol 54: 774-7, 2001.

78) Yoshimura M, Isomoto H, Shikuwa S, Osabe M, Matsunaga K, Omagari K, . Kohno S. A case of acute gastric mucosal lesions associated with *Helicobacter heilmannii* infection. Helicobacter, 7: 322–326, 2002.

79) van Loon S, Bart A, den Hertog EJ, Nikkels PG, Houwen RH, De Schryver JE, Oudshoorn JH. *Helicobacter heilmannii* gastritis caused by cat to child transmission. J Pediatr Gastroenterol Nutr 36: 407-9, 2003.

80) Boyanova L, Koumanova R,Lazarova E, Jelev C. *Helicobacter pylori* and *Helicobacter heilmannii* in children. A Bulgarian study. Diagn Microbiol Infect Dis 46:249-52, 2003.

81) Wooten DC, Rakheja D, Timmons CF. *Helicobacter heilmannii* infection in a child. Arch Pathol Lab Med 128:1461-2, 2004.

82) Sýkora J, Hejda V, Varvarovská J, Stozický F, Siala K, Schwarz J. *Helicobacter heilmannii* gastroduodenal disease and clinical aspects in children with dyspeptic symptoms. Acta Paediatr. 93:707-9, 2004.

83) Okiyama Y, Matsuzawa K, Hidaka E, Sano K, Akamatsu T, Ota H. *Helicobacter heilmannii* infection: Clinical, endoscopic and histopathological features in Japanese patients. Pathol Int 55: 398-404, 2005.

84) Kato S, Ozawa K, Sekine H, Ohyauchi M, Shimosegawa T, Minoura T, Iinuma K. *Helicobacter heilmannii* infection in a child after successful eradication of *Helicobacter pylori*: case report and review of literature. J Gastroenterol 40: 94-7, 2005.

85) Singhal AV, Sepulveda AR: *Helicobacter heilmannii* gastritis: a case study with review of literature. Am J Surg Pathol 29: 1537-9, 2005.

86) Orel R, Mlinaric V, Stepec S, Luzar B, Brencic E, Cerar A. Acute phlegmonous gastritis associated with *Helicobacter heilmannii* infection in a child. Dig Dis Sci 51: 2322-2325, 2006.

87) Oyauchi M, Ohara S, Sekine J, Shimosegawa T. A case of Barrett adenocaricinoma with Helicobacter heilmannii infection. Itocho, 41: 1089-1093, 2006 (in Japanese).

88) Siala K, Sykora J, He's O, Varvarovska J, Pandora P. *Helicobacter heilmannii* reinfection in a Helicobacter pylori negative adolescent: a 4-year follow-up. J Clin Gastroenterol 41: 221-222, 2007.

89) Qualia,CM, Katzman PJ, Brown MR & Kooros K. A report of two children with *Helicobacter heilmannii* gastritis and review of the literature. Pediatric and Developmental Pathology 10: 391–394, 2007.

90) Joo M, Kwak JE, Chang SH, Kim H, Chi JG, Kim K-A, Yang JH, Lee JS, Moon Y-S, Kim K-M. *Helicobacter heilmannii*-associated Gastritis: Clinicopathologic Findings and Comparison with *Helicobacter pylori*-associated Gastritis. J Korean Med Sci 22: 63-69, 2007.

91) Boyanova L, Lazarova E, Jelev C, Gergova G, Mitov I. *Helicobacter pylori* and *Helicobacter heilmannii* in untreated Bulgarian children over a period of 10 years. J Med Microbiol 56: 1081-1085, 2007.

92) Matsumoto, T., Kawakubo, M., Shiohara, M. *et al.* Phylogeny of a novel "*Helicobacter heilmannii*" organism from a Japanese patient with chronic gastritis based on DNA sequence analysis of 16S rRNA and urease genes. J Microbiol 47: 201–207, 2009.

93) Jothimani DK, Zanetto U, Owen RJ, Lawson AJ, Wilson PG. An unusual case of gastric erosions. Gut 58:1669, 1708, 2009.

94) Iwanczak B, Biernat M, Iwanczak F, Grabinska J, Matusiewicz K, Gosciniak G. The clinical aspects of *Helicobacter heilmannii* infection in children with dyspeptic symptoms. J Physiol Pharmacol 63:133-6, 2012.

95) Ohtaka M, Tatsumi A, Fukasawa M, Yamaguchi T, Uetake T, Ohtska H, Sato T, Enomoto N, Watanabe H, Mitani K. Complete remission of gastric plasmacytoma following eradication of '*Candidatus* Helicobacter heilmannii'. Clin J Gastroenterol 5:158–163, 2012.

96) Okamura T, Iwaya Y, Yokosawa S, Suga T, Arakura N, Matsumoto T, Ogiwara N, Higuchi K, Ota H, Tanaka E. A case of *Helicobacter heilmannii*-associated primary gastric mucosa-associated lymphoid tissue lymphoma achieving complete remission after eradication. Clin J Gastroenterol, 6: 38-45, 2013.

97) Liu J, He L, Haesebrouck F, Gong Y, Flahou B, Cao Q, Zhang J. Prevalence of Coinfection with Gastric Non-*Helicobacter pylori* Helicobacter (NHPH) Species in *Helicobacter pylori*-infected Patients Suffering from Gastric Disease in Beijing, China. Helicobacter 20: 284-90, 2015.

98) Matsumoto T, Kawakubo M, Akamatsu T, Koide N, Ogiwara N, Kubota S, Sugano M, Kawakami Y, Katsuyama T, Ota H. *Helicobacter heilmannii sensu stricto*-related gastric ulcers: a case report. World J Gastroenterol 20: 3376-3382, 2014.

99) Goji S, Tamura Y, Sasaki M, Nakamura M, Matsui H, Murayama SY, Ebi M, Ogasawara N, Funaki Y & Kasugai K. *Helicobacter suis*-infected nodular gastritis and a review of diagnostic sensitivity for *Helicobacter heilmannii*-like organisms. Case reports in gastroenterology, 9: 179–187, 2015.

100) Shiratori S, Mabe K, Yoshii S, Takakuwa Y, Sato M, Nakamura M &Sakamoto N. Two cases of chronic gastritis with non-*Helicobacter pylori* helicobacter infection. Internal Medicine 55: 1865–1869, 2016.

101) Kobayashi M, Yamamoto K, Ogiwara N, Matsumoto T, Shigeto S, Ota H. *Helicobacter heilmannii*-like organism in parietal cells: A diagnostic pitfall. Pathol Int 66: 120-2, 2016.

102) Øverby A, Murayama SY, Michimae H, Suzuki H, Suzuki M, Serizawa H, Tamura R, Nakamura S, Takahashi S & Nakamura M. Prevalence of gastric non-*Helicobacter pylori*-Helicobacters in Japanese patients with gastric disease. Digestion 95: 61-66, 2017.

103) Tsukadaira T, Hayashi S, Ota Y, *et al.* Nine cases of NHPH in fected gastritis, with successful eradication by proton pump inhibitors. Japanese Journal of Helicobacter Research, 18: 21-27, 2017 (in Japanese).

104) Nakagawa S, Shimoyama T, Nakamura M, *et al.* The resolution of *Helicobacter suis*-associated gastric lesions after eradication therapy. Intern Med. Tokyo Jpn 57: 203-207, 2018.

105) Takigawa H, Masaki S, Naito T, Yuge R, Urabe Y, Tanaka S, Sentani K, Matsuo T, Matsuo K, Chayama K & Kitadai Y. *Helicobacter suis* infection is associated with nodular gastritis-like appearance of gastric mucosa-associated lymphoid tissue lymphoma. Cancer medicine 8: 4370–4379, 2019.

106) Suzuki S, Miyachi E, Murayama S, Nakamura M, Terao S. Four cases of non-*Helicobacter pylori* Helicobacter-infected gastritis in our hospital. Japanese Journal of Helicobacter Research, 20: 77-83, 2019 (in Japanese).

107) Nakamura M, Øverby A, Michimae H, *et al.* PCR analysis and specific immunohistochemistry revealing a high prevalence of non‐*Helicobacter pylori* Helicobacters in *Helicobacter pylori*‐negative gastric disease patients in Japan: High susceptibility to an Hp eradication regimen. Helicobacter 25: e12700, 2020.

108) Shafaie S, Kaboosi, H. & Peyravii Ghadikolaii, F. Prevalence of non-*Helicobacter pylori* gastric Helicobacters in Iranian dyspeptic patients. BMC Gastroenterol 20: 190, 2020.

109) Takemoto T, Mizuno Y. Endoscopic diagnosis of chronic gastritis and gastric biopsy. Gastroenterol Endosc 4: 310 - 320, 1962 (in Japanese).

110) Miyagawa H, Takechi K, Kato S, *et al.* Clinical and immunological studies on nodular gastritis. Gastroenterol Endosc 27: 1275 - 1279, 1985.

111) Czinn SJ, Dahms BB, Jacobs GH, *et al.* Campylobacter - like organisms in association with symptomatic gastritis in children. J Pediatr 109: 80 - 83, 1986.

112) Konno M, Muraoka T. Characteristics of pediatric *Helicobacter pylori*-induced gastritis. Helicobacter Research 3: 32 - 37, 1999 (in Japanese).

113) Kamada T, Inoue K, Mabe Y, *et al.* Jevenile *Helicobacter pylori* gastritis. Helicobacter Research 17: 564 - 569, 2013 (in Japanese).

114) Sugimitsu N, Harada N, Iwasa T, *et al.*: Two cases of juvenile undifferentiated gastric cancer associated with nodular gastritis. The Japanese Journal of Clinical and Experimental Medicine. 88: 1177 - 1180, 2010 (in Japanese).

115) Nakamura M, Takahashi T, Matsui H, *et al.* Formation of nodular gastritis and its relation to *Helicobacter heilmannii*-like organism. Prog Med 30: 781-78at al.3, 2010 (in Japanese).

116) Matsui H, Takahashi T, Murayama SY, *et al.* Development of new PCR primers by comparative genomics for the detection of *Helicobacter suis* in gastric biopsy specimens. Helicobacter 19: 260-271, 2014.

117) Sasaki M, Goji S, Tamura Y, *et al.* *Helicobacter suis*-infected nodular gastritis and a review of diagnostic sensitivity for Helicobacter heilmannii-like organisms. Case Rep Gastroenterol 9: 179-187, 2015.

118) Konjetzny GE. Entgunclungen des margens. Handbuch der speziellen pathologischen anatome and histologie. 4th Ed, Henke F, Lubarsch 0.Springer, Berlin, 1928: 768-1116

Chapter 5 Diagnostic methods for gastric NHPH

119) Fawcett PT, Gibney KM, Vinette KM. *Helicobacter pylori* can be induced to assume the morphology of *Helicobacter heilmannii.* J Clin Microbiol.37: 1045-8. 1999. doi: 10.1128/JCM.37.4.1045-1048.1999. PMID: 10074524; PMCID: PMC88647.

120) Lee A, Dent J, Hazell S, & McNulty C. Origin of spiral organisms in human gastric antrum. Lancet 1 (8580): 300-1,1988.

121) Andersen LP, Norgaard, A, Holck S, Blom J & Elsborg L. Isolation of a *Helicobacter heilmannii*-like organism from the human stomach. Eur. J. Clin. Microbiol. Infect Dis 15: 95-96, 1996.

122) Jalava K, On SLW, Harrington CS, Andersen LP, M. Hanninen L, and Vandamme P. A cultured strain of "*Helicobacter heilmannii*," a human gastric pathogen, identified as *H. bizzozeronii*: evidence for zoonotic potential of Helicobacter. Emerg. Infect. Dis. 7: 1036-1038, 2001.

123) Baele M, Decostere A, Vandamme P, Ceelen L, Hellemans A, Mast J, Chiers K, Ducatelle R, Haesebrouck F. Isolation and characterization of *Helicobacter suis* sp. nov. from pig stomachs. Int J Syst Evol Microbiol. 58(Pt 6):1350-8, 2008. doi: 10.1099/ijs.0.65133-0. PMID: 18523177.

124) Liang J, De Bruyne E, Ducatelle R, Smet A, Haesebrouck F & Flahou B. Purification of *Helicobacter suis* strains from biphasic cultures by single colony isolation: influence on strain characteristics. HELICOBACTER, 20: 206–216, 2015.

125) Nakamura M, Øverby A, Matsui H. Morphological studies on non -Helicobacter pylori Helicobacter by biphasic culture system. 23rd Japanese Helicobacter meeting in Hakodate. June 30 to July 02, 2017.

126) Rimbara E, Suzuki M, Matsui H, Nakamura M, Kobayashi H, Mori S, Shibayama K. Complete Genome Sequence of Helicobacter suis Strain SNTW101c, Originally Isolated from a Patient with Nodular Gastritis. Microbiol Resour Announc. 9(1): e01340-19, 2020. doi: 10.1128/MRA.01340-19. PMID: 31896646; PMCID: PMC6940298.

Chapter 6 Elucidation of the phylogenetic tree and genome of NHPH

127) Trebesius K, Adler K, Vieth M, *et al.* Specific detection and prevalence of *Helicobacter heilmannii*-like organisms in the human gastric mucosa by fluorescent *in situ* hybridization and partial 16S ribosomal DNA sequencing. J Clin Microbiol 39: 1510-1516, 2001.

128) Chisholm SA, Owen RJ. Development and application of a novel screening PCR assay for direct detection of '*Helicobacter heilmannii*'-like organisms in human gastric biopsies in Southeast England. Diagn Microbiol Infect Dis 46: 1-7, 2003.

129) O'Rourke JL, Solnick JV, Neilan BA, *et al.* Description of "*Candidatus* Helicobacter heilmannii" based on DNA sequence analysis of 16S rRNA and urease genes. Int J Syst Evol Microbiol 54(Pt 6): 2203-2211, 2004.

130) Vermoote M, Vandekerckhove TTM, Flahou B, *et al.* Genome sequence of *Helicobacter suis* supports its role in gastric pathology. Vet Res 42: 51, 2011.

131) Arnold IC, Zigova Z, Holden M, *et al.* Comparative whole genome sequence analysis of the carcinogenic bacterial model pathogen *Helicobacter felis*. Genome Biol Evol 3: 302-308, 2011.

132) Schott T, Rossi M, Hänninen M-L. Genome sequence of *Helicobacter bizzozeronii* strain CIII-1, an isolate from human gastric mucosa. J Bacteriol 193: 4565-4566, 2011.

133)Smet A, Van Nieuwerburgh F, Ledesma J, *et al.* Genome sequence of *Helicobacter heilmannii sensu stricto* ASB1 isolated from the gastric mucosa of a kitten with severe gastritis. Genome Announc 1(1): e00033-12, 2013.

134) Matsui H, Takahashi T, Murayama SY, Uchiyama I, Yamaguchi K, Shigenobu S, Matsumoto T, Kawakubo M, Horiuchi K, Ota H, Osaki T, Kamiya S, Smet A, Flahou B, Ducatelle R, Haesebrouck F, Takahashi S, Nakamura S, Nakamura M. Development of new PCR primers by comparative genomics for the detection of *Helicobacter suis* in gastric biopsy specimens. Helicobacter 19:260-71, 2014. doi: 10.1111/hel.12127. Epub 2014 Mar 28. PMID: 24673878.

135) Joosten M, Linden S, Rossi M, *et al.* Divergence between the highly virulent zoonotic pathogen *Helicobacter heilmannii* and its closest relative, the low-virulence "*Helicobacter ailurogastricus*" sp. nov. Infect Immun 84, 293-306, 2015.

136) Cao DM, Lu QF, Li SB, Wang JP, Chen YL, Huang YQ, Bi HK. Comparative Genomics of H. pylori and Non-*Pylori* Helicobacter Species to Identify New Regions Associated with Its Pathogenicity and Adaptability. Biomed Res Int. 2016:6106029. doi: 10.1155/2016/6106029. Epub 2016 Dec 18. PMID: 28078297; PMCID: PMC5203880.

137) Shen Z, Mannion A, Lin M, Esmail M, Bakthavatchalu V, Yang S, Ho C, Feng Y, Smith B, Elliott J, Gresham V, VandeBerg JL, Samollow PB, Fox JG. *Helicobacter monodelphidis sp. nov.* and *Helicobacter didelphidarum sp. nov.*, isolated from grey short-tailed opossums (Monodelphis domestica) with endemic cloacal prolapses. Int J Syst Evol Microbiol. 70:6032-6043, 2020. doi: 10.1099/ijsem.0.004424. PMID: 33079029.

138) Hu S, Niu L, Wu L, Zhu X, Cai Y, Jin D, Yan L, Zhao F. Genomic analysis of *Helicobacter himalayensis* sp. nov. isolated from Marmota himalayana. BMC Genomics. 21:826, 2020. doi: 10.1186/s12864-020-07245-y. PMID: 33228534; PMCID: PMC7685656.

139) Gruntar I, Papić B, Pate M, Zajc U, Ocepek M, Kušar D. *Helicobacter labacensis* sp. nov., *Helicobacter mehlei sp. nov.*, and *Helicobacter vulpis sp. nov.*, isolated from gastric mucosa of red foxes (Vulpes vulpes). Int J Syst Evol Microbiol. 70: 2395-2404, 2020. doi: 10.1099/ijsem.0.004050. Epub 2020 Feb 18. PMID: 32068523.

140) Rimbara E, Suzuki M, Matsui H, Nakamura M, Kobayashi H, Mori S, Shibayama K. Complete Genome Sequence of *Helicobacter suis* Strain SNTW101c, Originally Isolated from a Patient with Nodular Gastritis. Microbiol Resour Announc. 9: e01340-19, 2020. doi: 10.1128/MRA.01340-19. PMID: 31896646; PMCID: PMC6940298.

141) Chan WS, Au CH, Leung HC, Ho DN, Chan TL, Lam TW, Ma ES, Tang BS. Draft Genome Sequence of *Helicobacter cinaedi*, Compiled by Direct Whole-Genome Sequencing of a Blood Culture-Positive Isolate in Hong Kong. Microbiol Resour Announc. 7: e01263-18, 2018. doi: 10.1128/MRA.01263-18. PMID: 30533780; PMCID: PMC6256545.

142) Shen Z, Batac F, Mannion A, Miller MA, Bakthavatchalu V, Ho C, Manning S, Paster BJ, Fox JG. Novel urease-negative Helicobacter sp. '*H. enhydrae sp. nov.*' isolated from inflamed gastric tissue of southern sea otters. Dis Aquat Organ. 123:1-11, 2017. doi: 10.3354/dao03082. PMID: 28177288.

143) Shen Z, Feng Y, Muthupalani S, Sheh A, Cheaney LE, Kaufman CA, Gong G, Paster BJ, Fox JG. Novel Helicobacter species *H. japonicum* isolated from laboratory mice from Japan induces typhlocolitis and lower bowel carcinoma in C57BL/129 IL10-/- mice. Carcinogenesis. 37:1190-1198, 2016. doi: 10.1093/carcin/bgw101. Epub 2016 Sep 21. PMID: 27655833; PMCID: PMC5137264.

144) Shen Z, Mannion A, Whary MT, Muthupalani S, Sheh A, Feng Y, Gong G, Vandamme P, Holcombe HR, Paster BJ, Fox JG. Helicobacter saguini, a Novel Helicobacter Isolated from Cotton-Top Tamarins with Ulcerative Colitis, Has Proinflammatory Properties and Induces Typhlocolitis and Dysplasia in Gnotobiotic IL-10-/- Mice. Infect Immun. 84(8): 2307-2316, 2016. doi: 10.1128/IAI.00235-16. PMID: 27245408; PMCID: PMC4962630.

145) Frank J, Dingemanse C, Schmitz AM, Vossen RH, van Ommen GJ, den Dunnen JT, Robanus-Maandag EC, Anvar SY. The Complete Genome Sequence of the Murine Pathobiont *Helicobacter typhlonius*. Front Microbiol.6: 1549, 2016. doi: 10.3389/fmicb.2015.01549. PMID: 26779178; PMCID: PMC4705304.

146) Walter J, Ley R. The human gut microbiome: ecology and recent evolutionary changes. Annu Rev Microbiol. 65: 411-29, 2011. doi: 10.1146/annurev-micro-090110-102830. PMID: 21682646.

147) Mannion A, Shen Z, Fox JG. Comparative genomics analysis to differentiate metabolic and virulence gene potential in gastric versus enterohepatic Helicobacter species. BMC Genomics. 19(1): 830, 2018. doi: 10.1186/s12864-018-5171-2. PMID: 30458713; PMCID: PMC6247508.

148) Maurer KJ, Ihrig MM, Rogers AB, Ng V, Bouchard G, Leonard MR, Carey MC, Fox JG. Identification of cholelithogenic enterohepatic helicobacter species and their role in murine cholesterol gallstone formation. Gastroenterology 128: 1023-33, 2005. doi: 10.1053/j.gastro.2005.01.008. PMID: 15825083.

149) Belzer C, Kusters JG, Kuipers EJ, van Vliet AH. Urease induced calcium precipitation by Helicobacter species may initiate gallstone formation. Gut 55:1678-9, 2006. doi: 10.1136/gut.2006.098319. PMID: 17047128; PMCID: PMC1860090.

150) Flahou B, Bakker MR, Langermans JAM, *et al.*: Evidence for a primate origin of zoonotic *Helicobacter suis* colonizing domesticated pigs. The ISME J (8 September 2017) | doi: 10.1038/ismej. 2017. 145

151) De Witte C, Berlamont H, Smet A, Ducatelle R, Haesebrouck F. Rhesus macaques are most likely the ancestral source of *Helicobacter suis* infection in pigs and not cynomolgus macaques. Helicobacter. 25:e12689, 2020. doi: 10.1111/hel.12689. Epub 2020 Mar 26. PMID: 32219893.

152) Berlamont H, Smet A, De Bruykere S, Boyen F, Ducatelle R, Haesebrouck F, De Witte C. Antimicrobial susceptibility pattern of *Helicobacter suis* isolates from pigs and macaques. Vet Microbiol. 239: 108459, 2019. doi: 10.1016/j.vetmic.2019.108459. Epub 2019 Nov 2. PMID: 31767067.

153) Smet A, Yahara K, Rossi M, Tay A, Backert S, Armin E, Fox JG, Flahou B, Ducatelle R, Haesebrouck F, Corander J. Macroevolution of gastric Helicobacter species unveils interspecies admixture and time of divergence. ISME J. 12:2518-2531, 2018. doi: 10.1038/s41396-018-0199-5. Epub 2018 Jun 25. Erratum in: ISME J. 2019 Feb 28;: PMID: 29942073; PMCID: PMC6154992.

Chapter 7 Bacterial eradication

154) Guidelines of diagnosis and treatment of H. pylori infection. 2016, by Guideline Committee of Japanese Helicobacter Society.Sentanigakusha (in Japanese).

Chapter 8 Clinical reports from Japan

Chapter 9 The examination of gastric NHPH with experimental models, especially gastric MALT lymphoma

155) Burkitt MD, Duckworth CA, Williams JM, Pritchard DM. *Helicobacter pylori*-induced gastric pathology: insights from in vivo and ex vivo models. Dis Model Mech.10(2):89-104, 2017. doi: 10.1242/dmm.027649. PMID: 28151409; PMCID: PMC5312008.

156)Enno A, O'Rourke JL, Howlett CR, Jack A, Dixon MF, Lee A. MALToma-like lesions in the murine gastric mucosa after long-term infection with *Helicobacter felis*. A mouse model of *Helicobacter pylori*-induced gastric lymphoma. Am J Pathol 147: 217-22, 1995. PMID: 7604881; PMCID: PMC1869885.

157) Erdman, S.E., Correa, P., Coleman, L.A., Schrenzel, M.D., Li, X. and Fox, J.G. *Helicobacter mustelae*-associated gastric MALT lymphoma in ferrets. Am J Pathol 151: 273-280, 1997.

158) Enno A, O'Rourke J, Braye S, Howlett R, Lee A. Antigen-dependent progression of mucosa-associated lymphoid tissue (MALT)-type lymphoma in the stomach. Effects of antimicrobial therapy on gastric MALT lymphoma in mice. Am J Pathol 152: 1625-1632, 1998.

159) Dieterich C, Bouzourene H, Blum AL and Corthesy-Theulaz IE. Urease-based mucosal immunization against *Helicobacter heilmannii* infection induces corpus atrophy in mice. Infect Immun., 67: 6206-6209, 1999.

160) Park, J.H., Seok, S.H., Baek, M.W., Lee, H.Y., Kim, D.J. and Park, J.H. Gastric lesions and immune responses caused by long-term infection with *Helicobacter heilmannii* in C57BL/6 mice. J Comp Pathol 139: 208-217, 2008.

161) O'Rourke JL, Dixon MF, Jack A, Enno A, Lee A. Gastric B-cell mucosa-associated lymphoid tissue (MALT) lymphoma in an animal model of '*Helicobacter heilmannii*' infection. J Pathol. 203: 896-903, 2004. doi: 10.1002/path.1593. PMID: 15258991.

162) Fukui T, Okazaki K, Tamaki H, et al. Immunogenetic analysis of gastric MALT lymphoma-like lesions induced by *Helicobacter pylori* infection in neonatally thymectomized mice. Lab Invest 84: 485-492, 2004.

163) Hellemans A, Decostere A, Haesebrouck F, Ducatelle R. Evaluation of antibiotic treatment against "*Candidatus* Helicobacter suis" in a mouse model. Antimicrob Agents Chemother. 49: 4530-5, 2005. doi:10.1128/AAC.49.11.4530-4535.2005. PMID: 16251292; PMCID: PMC1280154.

164) Hellemans A, Decostere A, Duchateau L, De Bock M, Haesebrouck F, Ducatelle R. Protective immunization against "Candidatus Helicobacter suis" with heterologous antigens of H. pylori and H. felis. Vaccine. 24: 2469-76. doi: 10.1016/j.vaccine.2005.12.033. Epub 2006 Jan 4. PMID: 16423431.

165) Nakamura M, Murayama SY, Serizawa H, *et al.* "Candidatus Helicobacter heilmannii" from a cynomolgus monkey induces gastric mucosa-associated lymphoid tissue lymphomas in C57BL/6 mice. Infect Immun 75: 1214-1222, 2007.

166) Nishikawa, K., Nakamura, M., Takahashi, S., *et al.* Increased apoptosis and angiogenesis in gastric low-grade mucosa- associated lymphoid tissue-type lymphoma by Helicobacter heilmannii infection in C57/BL6 mice. FEMS Immunol Med Microbiol 50, 268-272, 2007.

167) Nakamura M, Takahashi S, Matsui H, *et al.* Microcirculatory alteration in low-grade gastric mucosa-associated lymphoma by Helicobacter heilmannii infection: its relation to vascular endothelial growth factor and cyclooxygenase-2. Journal of Gastroenterology and Hepatology. 23 Suppl 2:S157-60, 2008. DOI: 10.1111/j.1440-1746.2008.05554.x.

168) Park JH, Seok SH, Baek MW, Lee HY, Kim DJ, Park JH. Gastric lesions and immune responses caused by long-term infection with Helicobacter heilmannii in C57BL/6 mice. J Comp Pathol. 139: 208-17, 2008. doi: 10.1016/j.jcpa.2008.04.005. Epub 2008 Sep 26. PMID: 18823636.

169) Matsui H, Aikawa C, Sekiya Y, Takahashi S, Murayama SY, Nakamura M. Evaluation of antibiotic therapy for eradication of "Candidatus Helicobacter heilmannii". Antimicrob Agents Chemother 2008 Aug;52: 2988-9. doi: 10.1128/AAC.01662-07. Epub May 19, 2008. PMID: 18490502; PMCID: PMC2493118.

170) Nakamura M, Matsui H, Takahashi T, Ogawa S, Tamura R, Murayama SY, Takahashi S, Tsuchimoto K. Suppression of lymphangiogenesis induced by Flt-4 antibody in gastric low-grade mucosa-associated lymphoid tissue lymphoma by Helicobacter heilmannii infection. J Gastroenterol Hepatol. 25 Suppl 1:S1-6, 2010. doi: 10.1111/j.1440-1746.2010.06230.x. PMID: 20586849.

171) Flahou B, Haesebrouck F, Pasmans F, D'Herde K, Driessen A, Van Deun K, Smet A, Duchateau L, Chiers K, Ducatelle R. Helicobacter suis causes severe gastric pathology in mouse and mongolian gerbil models of human gastric disease. PLoS One. 22;5: e14083, 2010. doi: 10.1371/journal.pone.0014083. PMID: 21124878; PMCID: PMC2989923.

172) Suzuki A, Kobayashi M, Matsuda K, *et al.* Induction of high endothelial venule-like vessels expressing GlcNAc6ST-1- mediated L-selectin ligand carbohydrate and mucosal addressin cell adhesion molecule 1 (MAdCAM-1) in a mouse model of "Candidatus Helicobacter heilmannii"- induced gastritis and gastric mucosa-associated lymphoid tissue (MALT) lymphoma. Helicobacter 15: 538-548, 2010.

173) Nobutani K, Yoshida M, Nishiumi S, Nishitani Y, Takagawa T, Tanaka H, Yamamoto K, Mimura T, Bensuleiman Y, Ota H, Takahashi S, Matsui H, Nakamura M, Azuma T. Helicobacter heilmannii can induce gastric lymphoid follicles in mice via a Peyer's patch-independent pathway. FEMS Immunol Med Microbiol 60: 156-64, 2010. doi: 10.1111/j.1574-695X.2010.00731.x. Epub 2010 Sep 16. PMID: 20846360.

174) Nakamura M, Øverby A, Uehara A, Oda M, Takahashi S, Murayama SY and Matsui H. Significance of cholinergic and peptidergic nerves in stress-induced ulcer and MALT lymphoma formation. Curr Pharm Des 2017 Feb 10. doi: 10.2174/1381612823666170210144750. [Epub ahead of print]

175) Ayala GE, Dai H, Powell M, *et al.* Cancer-related axonogenesis and neurogenesis in prostate cancer. Clin Cancer Res 14: 7593-7603, 2008.

176) Shah N, Khurana S, Cheng K, *et al:* Muscarinic receptors and ligands in cancer. Am J Physiol Cell Physiol 296: C221-C232, 2009.

177) Erin N, Duymus O, Ozturk S, *et al.* Activation of vagal nerve by semapimod alters substance P levels and decreases breast cancer metastasis. Regul Pept 179: 101-8, 2012.

178) Zhao CM, Hayakawa Y, Kodama Y, *et al.* Denervation suppresses gastric tumorigenesis. Sci Transl Med 20: 250ra115, 2014.

179) Kodama Y, Sakaki K, Murasato F, *et al.* MALT lymphoma, stress ulcer and cholinergic nerves from the viewpoint of bilateral and unilateral truncal vagotomy and substance P. Curr Pharm Des 24; 1961-1965, 2018.

180) Erin N, Duymus O, Ozturk S, *et al*. Activation of values nerve by semapimod alters substance P levels and decreases breast cancer metastasis. Regul Pept 179: 101-108, 2012.

Chapter 10 The association with diseases other than in the digestive tract

181) Nakamura M, Kodama Y, Øverby A, Takahashi S, Ohshima K, Suzuki H, Murayama SY, Matsui H. *Helicobacter suis* infection in mouse induced not only gastric, but hepatic and pulmonary MALT lymphoma: relation to substance P. Curr Pharm Des. 26: 3039-3045, 2020.

182) Mattar WE, Alex BK, Sherker AH: Primary hepatic Burkitt lymphoma presenting with liver failure. Gastrointest Cancer 41: 261-263, 2010.

183) Aozasa K, Mishima K and Ohsawa M. Primary malignant lymphoma of the liver. Leuk Lymphoma 10: 353-357, 1993.

184) Enzan H. Primary hepatic malignant lymphoma. Kanzou, 41:85–89, 2000 (in Japanese).

185) Ohsawa M, Tomita Y, Hashimoto M, *et al*: Hepatitis C viral genome in a subset of primary hepatic lymphoma. Mod Pathol 11: 471-478, 1998

186) Nakamura M, Takahashi T, Matsui H, *et al.* Alteration of angiogenesis in *Helicobacter heilmannii*-induced mucosa-associated lymphoid tissue lymphoma: interaction with c-Met and hepatocyte growth factor. J Gastroenterol Hepatol 29 (Suppl 4): 70-76, 2014.

187) Piao J, Jeong J, Jung Jihyun, *et al*. Substance P promotes liver sinusoidal endothelium-mediated hepatic regeneration by NO/HGF regulation. J Interferon Cytokine Res 39: 147-154, 2019.

188) Wan Y, Meng F, Wu N, *et al*. Substance P increases liver fibrosis by differential changes I senescence of chlangiocytes and hepatic stellate cells. Hepatology 66: 528-541, 2017.

189) Bi L, Li J, Dan W, *et al*. Pulmonary MALT lymphoma; a case report and review of the literature. Ext Ther Med 9: 147-150, 2015.

190）Kodama Y, Sakaki K, Murasato F, *et al*. MALT lymphoma, stress ulcer and cholinergic nerves from the viewpoint of bilateral and unilateral truncal vagotomy and substance P. Curr Pharm Des 24; 1961-1965, 2018.

191) Munos M, González-Ortega A, Rosso M, *et al*. The substance P/neurokinin-1 receptor system in lung cancer: Focus on the antitumor action of neurokinin-1 receptor antagonists. Peptides 38: 318-325, 2010.

192))Iida T, Iwahashi M, Nakamura M, *et al*. Primary hepatic low-grade B-cell lymphoma of MALT-type associated with *Helicobacter pylori* infection. Hepatogastroenterology 54: 1898-1901, 2013.

193) Dong H, Chen L, Chen Y, *et al.* Primary hepatic extranodal marginal zone B-cell lymphoma of mucosa-associated lymphoid tissue type a case report and literature review. Medicine 96: e6305, 2017.

194) Yanai S, Nakai K, Tokuhara K, *et al.* A case of gastric MALT lymphoma discovered through pulmonary lesions. J Jpn Surg Assoc 70: 1970-1974, 2009.

Chapter 11 Cats and dogs as pets, pigs as livestock and gastric NHPH

195) Stolte M, Wellens E, Bethke B, Ritter M & Eidt H. *Helicobacter heilmannii* (formerly *Gastrospirillum hominis*) gastritis: an infection transmitted by animals? Scand J Gastroenterol 29: 1061-1064, 1994.

196)Meining A, Kroher G, & Stolte M. Animal reservoirs in the transmission of *Helicobacter heilmannii.* Results of a questionnaire-based study. Scandinavian journal of gastroenterology, 33: 795-8, 1998.

197) Eaton KA, Dewhirst FE, Paster BJ, *et al.* Prevalence and varieties of Helicobacter species in dogs from random sources and pet dogs: animal and public health implications. J Clin Microbiol 34:3165-3170, 1996. doi:10.1128/JCM.34.12.3165-3170.1996.

198) Serna JH, Genta RM, Lichtenberger LM, Graham DY, el-Zaatari FA. Invasive Helicobacter-like organisms in feline gastric mucosa. Helicobacter. 2:40-43, 1997. doi: 10.1111/j.1523-5378.1997.tb00056.x. PMID: 9432321.

199) Neiger R, Dieterich C, Burnens A, Waldvogel A, Corthesy-Theulaz I, Halter F, Lauterburg B, Schmassmann A: Detection and prevalence of Helicobacter infection in pet cats. J Clin Microbiol 36: 634-637, 1998.

200) De Groote D, Ducatelle R, van Doorn LJ, Tilmant K, Verschuuren A, Haesebrouck F. Detection of "*Candidatus* Helicobacter suis" in gastric samples of pigs byD PCR: comparison with other invasive diagnostic techniques. J Clin Microbiol 38: 1131-5, 2000. doi: 10.1128/JCM.38.3.1131-1135.2000. PMID: 10699008; PMCID: PMC86356.

201) Priestnall SL, Wiinberg B, Spohr A, Neuhaus B, Kuffer M, Wiedmann M, Simpson KW. Evaluation of "*Helicobacter heilmannii*" subtypes in the gastric mucosa of cats and dogs. J Clin Microbiol 42:2144-51, 2004. doi: 10.1128/jcm.42.5.2144-2151.2004. PMID: 15131182; PMCID: PMC404595.

202) Van den Bulck K, Baele M, Hermans K, Ducatelle R, Haesebrouck F & Decostere A. First report on the occurrence of "*Helicobacter heilmannii*" in the stomach of rabbits. Vet Res Commun 29: 271-27, 2005.

203) Ramis G, Gómez S, Pallarés FJ, Antonio Muñoz A. Prevalence of Helicobacter-like bacteria in the gastric mucosa of pigs slaughtered in south-east Spain. An Vet 23: 75-86, 2007.

204) Foss DL, Kopta LA, Paquette JA, Bowersock TL, et al. Identification of *Helicobacter suis* in pig-producing regions of the United States. J Swine Health Production 21: 242-247, 2013.

205) De Cooman L, Flahou B, Houf K, Smet A, Ducatelle R, Pasmans F, Haesebrouck F. Survival of *Helicobacter suis* bacteria in retail pig meat. Int J Food Microbiol 16;166: 164-7, 2013. doi: 10.1016/j.ijfoodmicro.2013.05.020. Epub 2013 Jun 6. PMID: 23880243.

206) MacHugh DE, Larson G, Orlando L. Taming the Past: Ancient DNA and the Study of Animal Domestication. Annu Rev Anim Biosci. 2017 Feb 8;5:329-351, 2017.

Authors' Biography

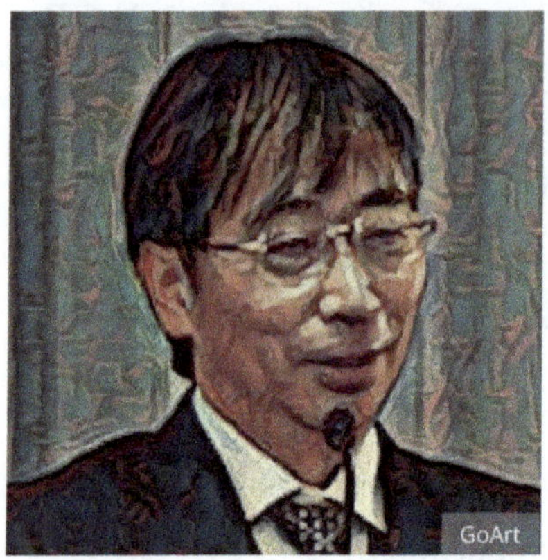

Masahiko NAKAMURA

Researcher, Satoshi Omura Memorial Institute, Kitasato University

-Formerly Associate Professor, School of Pharmacy, Kitasato University

-MD and PhD (Keio University)

-Speciality: Gastroenterology, Internal Medicine

-Areas of Interest: Autonomic nerves, Microcirculation and *Helicobacter heilmannii* (NHPH) in Gastric Mucosa

-Using mac from IIcx, 1989

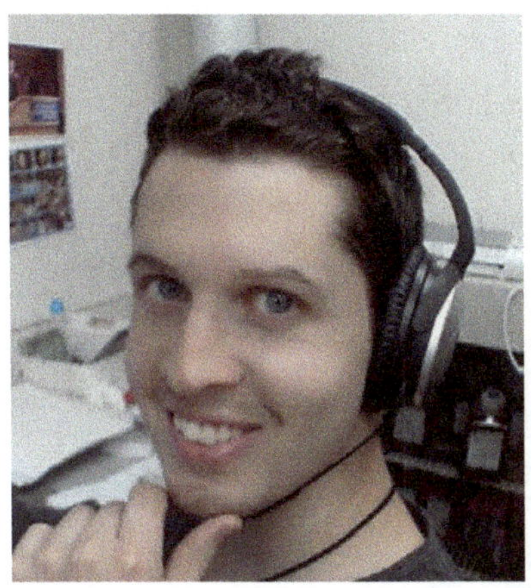

Anders ØVERBY

BSc and MSc in biotechnology

- PhD in molecular biology (NTNU Norway), focusing on gastric cancer

- 2 years as postdoctoral fellow at Kitasato University, School of pharmacy in Japan

- Experience with microbiology in an industrial/applied setting

- Fascinated by the occurrence of NHPH with respect to their nature, different species, zoonosis, prevalence and epidemiology

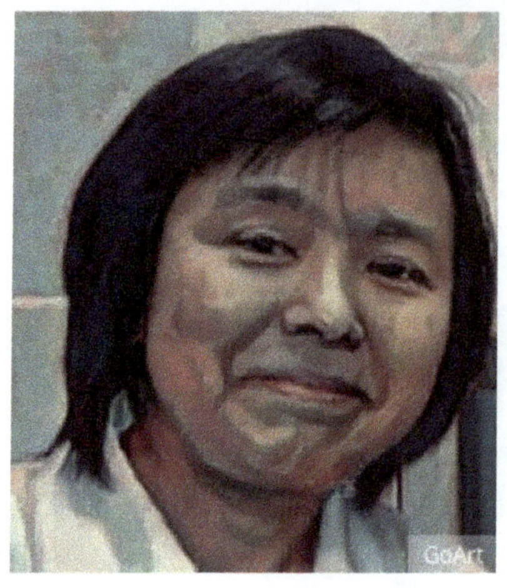

Somay Y MURAYAMA

Professor, School of Pharmacy, Nihon University

-PhD (Dr of Pharmacy, Chiba University)

-Speciality: Mycology

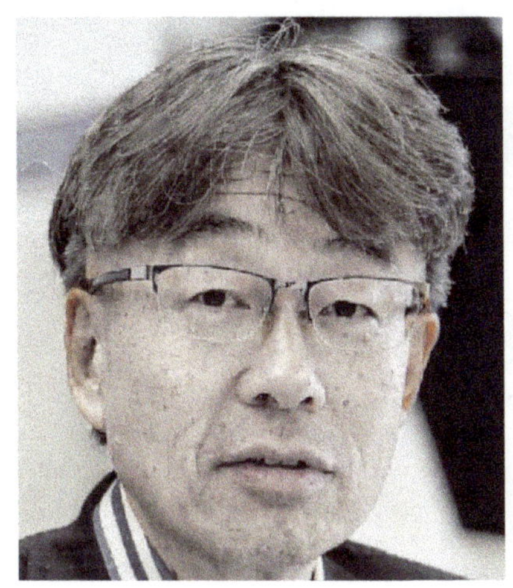

Hidekazu SUZUKI

-MD, PhD, FACG, RFF Professor, Department of Gastroenterology and Hepatology, Tokai University School of Medicine

-Speciality: Gastroenterology

-Area of Interest:

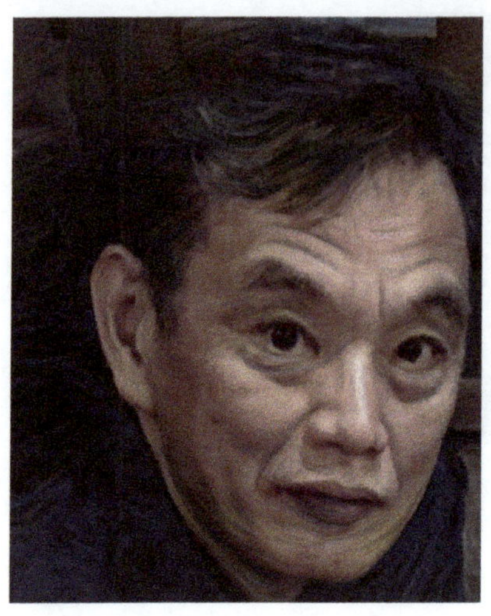

Hidenori MATSUI

Assistant Professor, Satoshi Omura Memorial Institute,
Kitasato University

-PhD (Doctor of Pharmacy, Chiba University)

-Speciality: Bacteriology (Molecular Biology)

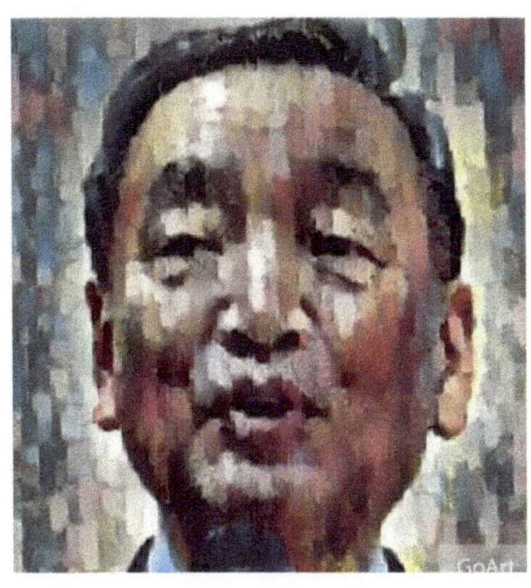

Shin'ichi TAKAHASHI

Deputy Director, Kosei Hospital

MD and PhD (Kyorin University)

-Formerly Professor, 3rd Dept of Internal Medicine, Kyorin University School of Medicine

-Speciality: Gastroenterology

Area of Interest: Helicobacter pylori

Non-Helicobacter pylori Helicobacter

-History, Biology and Disease

Second Edition

Publisher: Helicobacter heilmannii Study Group of Japan

URL http:heilmannii.versus.jp

June 2021

www.ingramcontent.com/pod-product-compliance
Ingram Content Group UK Ltd.
Pitfield, Milton Keynes, MK11 3LW, UK
UKHW021838270726
14058UKWH00002B/225

9 784991 166211